Midwifery Essentials
Basics

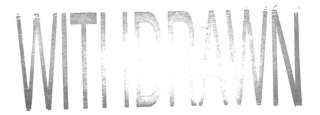

For Elsevier:

Commissioning Editor: Mairi McCubbin
Development Editor: Sheila Black
Project Manager: Christine Johnston
Designer: Charlotte Murray, Kirsteen Wright
Illustrations Manager: Merlyn Harvey

Midwifery Essentials
Volume 1 **Basics**

Helen Baston BA(Hons) MMedSci PhD ADM PGDipEd RN RM

Lead Midwife for Education; Supervisor of Midwives, Mother & Infant Research Unit, Department of Health Sciences, University of York, York, UK

Jennifer Hall MSc ADM PGDip(HE) RN RM

Senior Lecturer in Midwifery, Faculty of Health and Life Sciences, University of the West of England, Bristol, UK

Alyson Henley-Einion BSc(Hons) MA MAPD DipHE PGCE RN RM

Senior Lecturer in Midwifery, Faculty of Health and Life Sciences, University of the West of England, Bristol, UK

Foreword by
Mandy Renton BSc(Hons) MSc RN RM

General Manager, Peterborough and Stamford Hospitals NHS Foundation Trust, Peterborough, UK

With a contribution by
Anne-Marie Henshaw MMid RM RGN

Lecturer (Midwifery and Women's Health Group), Supervisor of Midwives, The School of Health Care, The University of Leeds, Leeds, UK

CHURCHILL LIVINGSTONE

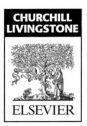

ELSEVIER

Edinburgh London New York Oxford Philadelphia St Louis Sydney Toronto 2009

CHURCHILL LIVINGSTONE
ELSEVIER

© 2009, Elsevier Limited. All rights reserved.

No part of this publication may be reproduced, stored in a retrieval system, or transmitted in any form or by any means, electronic, mechanical, photocopying, recording or otherwise, without the prior permission of the Publishers. Permissions may be sought directly from Elsevier's Health Sciences Rights Department, 1600 John F. Kennedy Boulevard, Suite 1800, Philadelphia, PA 19103-2899, USA: phone: (+1) 215 239 3804; fax: (+1) 215 239 3805; or, e-mail: *healthpermissions@elsevier. com*. You may also complete your request on-line via the Elsevier homepage (http://www.elsevier. com), by selecting 'Support and contact' and then 'Copyright and Permission'.

First published 2009
Reprinted 2009

ISBN 978-0-443-10353-7

British Library Cataloguing in Publication Data

A catalogue record for this book is available from the British Library

Library of Congress Cataloging in Publication Data

A catalog record for this book is available from the Library of Congress

Note

Knowledge and best practice in this field are constantly changing. As new research and experience broaden our knowledge, changes in practice, treatment and drug therapy may become necessary or appropriate. Readers are advised to check the most current information provided (i) on procedures featured or (ii) by the manufacturer of each product to be administered, to verify the recommended dose or formula, the method and duration of administration, and contraindications. It is the responsibility of the practitioner, relying on their own experience and knowledge of the patient, to make diagnoses, to determine dosages and the best treatment for each individual patient, and to take all appropriate safety precautions. To the fullest extent of the law, neither the Publisher nor the Editors assumes any liability for any injury and/or damage to persons or property arising out of or related to any use of the material contained in this book.

Working together to grow libraries in developing countries

www.elsevier.com | www.bookaid.org | www.sabre.org

ELSEVIER   **BOOK AID International**   **Sabre Foundation**

your source for books, journals and multimedia in the health sciences

www.elsevierhealth.com

The Publisher's policy is to use **paper manufactured from sustainable forests**

Printed in China

Contents

It seems a long time since I agreed to write a foreword for the first volume of this exciting new series of textbooks for student midwives and those who support them. My reason for agreeing to the request is the basis for this introductory note. I have always held a strong belief in the need for midwives to be strong academically and yet practical – able to apply their knowledge to their clinical care. I also have the utmost admiration for Helen Baston and Jennifer Hall for their commitment to the education and preparation of midwives both through their work as lecturers and also in the production of the 'Midwifery Basics' articles, which have become a regular and popular feature of *The Practising Midwife*.

Midwives need to be able to have confident, informed discussions with women and their families to both guide and empower them to make safe decisions in their pregnancy, birth and postnatal care. They must also be able to advocate for those women and for safe midwifery practice when discussing care and developing multidisciplinary policies and guidelines. All healthcare professionals involved in maternity service provision are aiming for the same outcome: a healthy and happy mother and baby.

It is my belief that in order to maintain the strength of support for women that is at the heart of midwifery practice, we must be knowledgeable, confident and up to date with the appropriate evidence to underpin the care we give. It is often our strong basic knowledge that enables us to progress debate and analyse complex issues. This text provides a comprehensive guide, covering basic skills such as taking a pulse or measuring blood pressure, so that students have a resource at hand that really meets their development needs.

Education of midwives is key to the future of the service. This is a great time for midwives to speak out and to take the maternity services forward in a way that will make a difference to women. We now have clear targets (Department of Health 2008) to help guide practice and service design – targets which really place women at the centre of care. Midwives must be in a position to steer developments through to success. In order to do that well, we must present ourselves in a way that promotes confidence to women, their families, our colleagues and health commissioners. This new series of books will have a valuable role in supporting midwives to take the maternity agenda forward.

Peterborough, 2009   Mandy Renton

Department of Health 2008 Maternity matters: choice, access and continuity of care in a safe service. Department of Health, London

To contribute to the provision of sensitive, safe and effective maternity care for women and their families is a privilege. Childbirth is a life-changing event for women. Those around them and those who input into any aspect of pregnancy, labour, birth or the postnatal period can positively influence how this event is experienced and perceived. In order to achieve this, maternity carers continually need to reflect on the services they provide and strive to keep up to date with developments in clinical practice. They should endeavour to ensure that women are central to the decisions made and that real choices are offered and supported by skilled practitioners.

This book is the first volume in a series of texts based on the popular 'Midwifery Basics' series published in *The Practising Midwife* journal. Since their publication, there have been many requests from students, midwives and supervisors to combine the articles into a handy text to provide a resource for learning and refreshment of midwifery knowledge and skills. The books have remained true to the original style of the articles and have been updated and expanded to create a user-friendly source of information. They are also intended to stimulate debate and require the reader both to reflect on their current practice, local policies and procedures and to challenge care that is not woman centred. The use of scenarios enables the practitioner to understand the context of maternity care and explore their role in its safe and effective provision.

There are many dimensions to the provision of woman-centred care that practitioners need to consider and understand. To aid this process, a jigsaw model has been introduced, with the aim of encouraging the reader to explore maternity care from a wide range of perspectives. For example, how does a midwife obtain consent from a woman for a procedure, maintain a safe environment during the delivery of care and make the most of the opportunity to promote health? What are the professional and legal issues in relation to the procedure and is this practice based on the best available evidence? Which members of the multi-professional team contribute to this aspect of care and how is it influenced by the way care is organized? Each aspect of the jigsaw should be considered during the assessment, planning, implementation and evaluation of woman-centred maternity care.

Midwifery Essentials: Basics is about learning to perform a range of clinical skills safely and with confidence. Each chapter is written to stand alone or be read in succession. The introductory chapter sets the scene, exploring the role of the midwife in the context of professional and national guidance. The jigsaw model for midwifery care is introduced and explained, providing a framework to explore the application of each of the clinical skills described in subsequent chapters. Central to undertaking each of the skills discussed is the need to communicate effectively with women and their families; this process is explored in Chapter 2. Effective communication is at the heart of the jigsaw model and is therefore explored throughout the book in relation to each of the clinical skills described. Chapter 3 introduces principles of infection control and how to assist women to meet their hygiene needs. Chapters 4, 5 and 6 cover the essential observations of blood pressure, temperature and pulse respectively. The next four chapters cover the collection of specimens, urinalysis, venepuncture and collection of blood from the woman and then the baby. Chapters 11 and 12 describe the principles of medicines management and injection technique. Finally,

Chapter 13 outlines the fundamentals of surgical care, which enable the reader to apply the knowledge gained in the preceding chapters. This book therefore prepares the reader to understand and master the basic clinical skills required for the provision of safe maternity care. Subsequent books in the series explore the principles and practice of contemporary antenatal, intrapartum and postnatal care, providing a comprehensive foundation for the care of women and their families throughout the childbirth continuum.

York and Bristol, 2009

Helen Baston
Jennifer Hall
Alyson Henley-Einion

Acknowledgements

In the process of writing there are always people behind the scenes who support or add to the development of the book. We would specifically like to thank Mary Seager, formerly Senior Commissioning Editor at Elsevier, for her initial vision, support and prompting to turn the journal articles from *The Practising Midwife* into a readable volume. We would also like to thank Anne-Marie Henshaw for her assistance in writing one of the chapters. Finally, none of us could have completed this project without the love, support, patience and endless cups of tea and coffee provided by our partners and children. To you we owe our greatest gratitude.

Chapter 1

Introduction

This book is the first in the *Midwifery Essentials* series aimed at student midwives and those who support them in clinical practice. This introductory chapter has two main aims:

- To describe the frameworks that support professional midwifery practice in the United Kingdom
- To introduce the 'jigsaw model' for exploring effective midwifery practice.

Both the frameworks and the model will be referred to throughout the book. The focus of this book is learning the skills relevant for midwifery practice. Although there will be reference to anatomy and physiology the reader will be directed to look in depth at the relevant systems of the body depending on the skill described.

The role of the midwife

Whether you are new to midwifery practice or in the process of updating your skills and knowledge it is important that you are fully aware of the remit of being a midwife. Many agencies contribute to the description of the midwife's position and together provide a comprehensive portfolio of the skills and attributes, knowledge and sphere of this complex role. The role of the midwife is however more than the sum of its constituent parts and many aspects of it evade measurement. For example, how can the intuition, emotional intelligence and sensitivity required for the development of a trusting relationship between a woman and her midwife be captured and formally assessed? Nevertheless, many aspects of the midwife's role have been identified and form the basis for professional guidance relating to educational programmes and subsequent clinical practice.

European Midwifery Directive

Midwives who work in the European Union (EU) must be able to fulfil the activities of a midwife as laid down in the European Union Second Midwifery Directive 80/155/EEC Article 4 and presented in the *Midwives rules and standards* (NMC 2004a); see Box 1.1.

Box 1.1 Activities of a midwife (NMC 2004a:36–37)

- To provide sound family planning information and advice
- To diagnose pregnancies and monitor normal pregnancies; to carry out examinations necessary for the monitoring of the development of normal pregnancies
- To prescribe or advise on the examinations necessary for the earliest possible detection of pregnancies at risk
- To provide a programme of parenthood preparation and complete preparation for childbirth, including advice on hygiene and nutrition
- To care for and assist the mother during labour and to monitor the condition of the fetus in utero by the appropriate clinical and technical means
- To conduct spontaneous deliveries including where required an episiotomy and in urgent cases, a breech delivery
- To recognize the warning signs of abnormality in the mother or infant which necessitate referral to a doctor and to assist the latter where appropriate; to take the necessary emergency measures in the doctor's absence, in particular the manual removal of the placenta, possibly followed by a manual examination of the uterus
- To examine and care for the newborn infant; to take all initiatives which are necessary in case of need and to carry out where necessary immediate resuscitation
- To care for and monitor the progress of the mother in the postnatal period and to give all necessary advice to the mother on infant care to enable her to ensure the optimal progress of the newborn infant
- To carry out treatment prescribed by a doctor
- To maintain all necessary records.

EU Second Midwifery Directive 80/155/EEC Article 4

Nursing and Midwifery Council

Midwives who work in the United Kingdom (UK) must be registered with the Nursing and Midwifery Council (NMC). The NMC is an organisation instituted by Parliament under the Nursing and Midwifery Order 2001 to protect the public by ensuring high standards of care are provided by nurses and midwives to their clients. To do this the NMC maintains a register of qualified nurses, midwives and specialist community public health nurses and set standards for practice and conduct. The NMC publishes standards regarding many aspects of professional practice and these are regularly reviewed. There are two that pertain specifically to midwifery: *Standards of proficiency for pre-registration midwifery education* (NMC 2004b) and the *Midwives rules and standards*, and many more that are generic to all registrants. Firstly, we will consider the *Standards of proficiency for pre-registration midwifery education*.

Standards of proficiency for pre-registration midwifery education

In addition to fulfilling the EU activities of a midwife, midwives in the UK must also demonstrate competence in the standards of proficiency for pre-registration midwifery education. These are the skills and practices that midwives should be competent to fulfil at the point of registration without direct supervision. They are presented in the NMC booklet *Standards of proficiency for pre-registration midwifery education* (NMC 2004b: 36–47) and form the basis for the assessment strategy for many pre-registration midwifery programmes. There are 29 midwifery proficiencies and they are described under four domains:

- Effective midwifery practice
- Professional and ethical practice
- Developing the individual midwife and others
- Achieving quality care through evaluation and research.

Each proficiency comprises a number of descriptors, for example, the proficiency 'communicate effectively' incorporates the descriptors, listening to women, enabling women to make their own choices, encouraging them to think through their feelings and should be demonstrated throughout the childbirth continuum of pregnancy to the postnatal period. A circular from the NMC identifies essential skills students should have learnt by different stages of their programmes (NMC 2007). Reference will be made to the midwifery proficiencies throughout this book to enable students and midwives to understand how they apply to clinical practice.

Midwives rules and standards

These are presented in the NMC booklet *Midwives rules and standards* (2004a) along with additional guidance on how they can be interpreted. They are the backbone of accountable midwifery practice in the UK and should be a well-thumbed resource in all midwives' personal profiles. The contents of *Midwives rules and standards* are summarized in Box 1.2.

Definition of the midwife
(Adopted by the International Confederation of Midwives Council 2005)

'A midwife is a person who, having been regularly admitted to a midwifery educational programme, duly recognized in the country in which it is located, has successfully completed the prescribed course of studies in midwifery and has acquired the requisite qualifications to be registered and/or legally licensed to practise midwifery.

The midwife is recognized as a responsible and accountable professional who works in partnership with women to give the necessary support, care and advice during pregnancy, labour and the postpartum period, to conduct births on the midwife's own responsibility and provide care for the newborn and the infant. This care includes preventative measures, the promotion of normal birth, the detection of complications in mother and child, the accessing of medical care or other appropriate assistance and the carrying out of emergency measures.

The midwife has an important task in health counselling and education, not only for the woman, but also within the family and the community. This work should involve antenatal education and preparation for parenthood and may extend to women's health, sexual or reproductive health and childcare.

Box 1.2 Midwives rules and standards (NMC 2004a)

Rule	Summary of content
1	How the rules should be cited and when they came into force
2	Interpretation of the rules: this section provides guidance on the meaning of some of the terms used throughout the rules, for example, what is meant by 'postnatal period'
3	Notification of intention to practise (NIP): how often and in what circumstances midwives should inform their local supervising authority (LSA) that they intend to practise midwifery in that locality
4	Notifications by local supervising authority: the people to whom and dates by which midwives should inform their intentions to practise above
5	Suspension from practice by a local supervising authority: the circumstances under and methods by which a midwife may be suspended from practice
6	Responsibility and sphere of practice: this section clearly outlines the role of the midwife
7	Administration of medicines: the responsibilities and guidance for a midwife in the administration of medicines
8	Clinical trials: the circumstances under which a midwife my participate in research trials
9	Records: the instructions and standards for record keeping
10	Inspection of premises and equipment: the rule governing the monitoring of equipment, premises and records by the local supervising authority
11	Eligibility for appointment as a supervisor of midwives: the rules governing the selection and training of supervisors of midwives
12	The supervision of midwives: instruction for the role of supervision
13	The local supervising authority midwifery officer: the role of the midwifery officer responsible for supervision in the locality
14	Exercise by a local supervising authority of its functions: the role of the LSA in supervision of the practice of the midwifery officer
15	Publication of local supervising authority procedures: the responsibilities of the LSA in giving information on those who have responsibility and dealing with complaints about processes and practices
16	Annual report : the responsibilities of the mechanisms of reporting by the LSA.

A midwife may practise in any setting including the home, community, hospitals, clinics or health units.'

The code of professional conduct

All nurses, midwives and public health specialists in the community are expected to adhere to a code of practice called *The Code. Standards of conduct, performance and ethics for nurses and midwives*. (NMC 2008) The standards have an underpinning principle of personal accountability for practice and of the value of the person being cared for. The code states that:

In caring for patients and clients, you must:

- Treat people as individuals and respect their confidentiality
- Collaborate with those in your care
- Ensure you gain consent and maintain clear professional boundaries
- Work effectively as part of a team, delegate effectively and manage risk
- Use the best evidence and keep your skills up to date
- Keep clear and accurate records
- Act with integrity, deal with problems, be impartial and uphold the reputation of your profession.

The role of the midwife therefore involves recognizing the worth and value of the individual.

National Service Framework (NSF)

The National Service Framework for Children, Young People and Maternity Services was published in 2004 by the Department of Health in the UK.

NSFs are government initiated long-term strategies. They:

- Set national standards and identify key interventions for a defined service or care group

- Put in place strategies to support implementation
- Establish ways to ensure progress within an agreed timescale
- Form one of a range of measures to raise quality and decrease variations in service. (See http://www.dh.gov.uk).

It presented a 10-year plan with the expectation that by 2014 the standards it introduced would be achieved. Standard 11 focused specifically on maternity services aiming to improve the care of mother and subsequently the unborn infant, and the long-term health of the child. The document recognized that for most women childbirth is a 'normal life event', and that improvement in the services would have a long-term effect on the child. Thus it is recognized that maternity care is important and that those who give the care are of value. Issues such as choice, continuity and woman-centred care are highlighted as relevant to women.

NICE guidelines

There are a range of clinical guidelines which have been produced after careful consideration of the available evidence by panels of experts in the field. Each guideline has a clear remit and offers best practice advice on the care of women and their babies. These NICE guidelines will be referred to throughout the book so that the reader can consider how local practice guidelines reflect national advice.

Midwifery care model

One of the purposes of this series is to consider the care of women and their babies from an holistic viewpoint. This means considering the care from a physical, emotional, psychological, spiritual, social and cultural context. To do this we have devised a jigsaw model

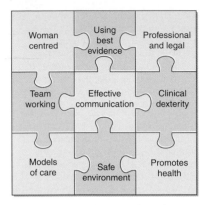

Fig. 1.1 Jigsaw model: dimensions of effective midwifery care.

of care that will encourage the reader to consider aspects of care, while recognizing these aspects to make up part of the whole person being cared for (Fig. 1.1).

This model will be used to reflect on the clinical scenarios described in the chapters. It shows the dimensions for effective maternity care and each should be considered during the assessment, planning, implementation and evaluation of an aspect of care.

The pieces of the jigsaw clearly interlink with each other and each is needed for the provision of safe, holistic care. When one is missing the picture will be incomplete and care will not reach its potential. Each aspect of the model is described below in more detail. It is recommended that when an aspect of midwifery care is being evaluated, each piece of the jigsaw is addressed. Consider the questions pertaining to each piece of the jigsaw and work through those that are relevant to the clinical situation you face.

Woman-centred care

The provision of woman-centred care was one of the central messages of the policy document *Changing Childbirth* (Department of Health 1993) which turned the focus of maternity care from meeting the needs of the professionals to listening and responding to the aspirations of women. This is further enforced in the NSF (2004) and is an expectation of midwifery education (NMC 2004b). When considering particular aspects of care the questions that need to be addressed to ensure that the woman's care is woman centred include:

- Was the woman involved in the development of her care plan and its subsequent implementation?
- Should her family or carers also need to be involved?
- How can I ensure that she remains involved in further decisions about her care?
- What are the implications of undertaking or not undertaking this procedure on this particular woman and baby?
- Are there any factors that I need to consider that might influence the results of this procedure for this woman and their impact on her?
- How does this procedure fit in with the woman's hopes and expectations?
- Is now the most appropriate time to undertake this procedure?

Using best evidence

The NMC code of professional conduct states 'you must deliver care based on the best evidence or best practice … ensure any advice you give is evidence based' (NMC 2008:07). Midwifery evidence includes many aspects (Wickham 2004) and the decisions a midwife makes about her practice will be influenced by a range of factors. However, in the statement above care should be based as much as possible on the 'best evidence', whatever that is.

Questions that need to be addressed to ensure that the woman's care is evidence based include:

- What is already known about this aspect of care?
- What is the research evidence available on this procedure?
- Do local guidelines reflect best evidence?
- What is the justification for the choices made about care?

Professional and legal

Midwives who practise in the United Kingdom must adhere to the rules and guidance of the Nursing and Midwifery Council (NMC). They are also required to comply with the law and the rules and regulations of the employers. Questions that need to be addressed to ensure that the woman's care fulfils statutory obligations include:

- Is this procedure expected to be an integral part of education prior to qualification?
- How do the midwives' rules relate to this procedure?
- Which NMC proficiencies relate to this procedure?
- How does the code of conduct relate to this procedure?
- Is there any other NMC guidance applicable to this procedure?
- Are there any national or international guidelines for this procedure?
- Are there any legal issues underpinning the use of this procedure?

Team working

Midwives work as part of a team of professionals who each bring particular skills and perspectives to the care of women and their families. The code of professional conduct requires registrants to 'work with others to protect and promote the health and wellbeing of those in your care, their families and carers, and the wider community' (NMC 2008:05). *Midwives rules and standards* also requires midwives to refer any woman or baby whose condition deviates from normal to an appropriate health professional (NMC 2004a:16).

Questions that need to be addressed to ensure that the woman's care makes appropriate use of the multi-professional team include:

- Does this procedure fall within my role?
- Who else will need to be involved to interpret the results?
- Where should these results be recorded for all to see?
- Whom will I involve if the results are outside normal parameters?
- How can I facilitate effective team working with this woman?
- Will another person be required to assist with this procedure?
- When will they be available?

Effective communication

Central to any interaction between a woman and the midwife is effective communication. It is essential that the midwife is aware of the cues she is giving to the woman during the care she provides. Time is often pressured in midwifery, both in the community and hospital setting but it is important to convey to the woman that she is the focus of your attention. Taking time to explain what you are going to do and why is crucial if she is going to trust that you are acting in her best interest. Questions that need to be addressed to ensure that effective communication is achieved before, during and after this procedure, include:

- What information needs to be given in order for the woman to choose whether this is the right procedure for her?

- Has she given consent?
- Is she clear what the procedure entails?
- In what ways could the information be given?
- What should be said during the procedure?
- What should be observed in the woman's behaviour during the procedure?
- What should be communicated to the woman after the procedure?
- How and where should recording of the procedure and its results be made?

Clinical dexterity

Midwifery is a profession that requires the practitioner to have a range of knowledge and a repertoire of clinical skills. The midwife continues to learn new skills throughout her working life and is accountable for maintaining and developing her practice as new ways of working are introduced (NMC 2008:07).

Questions that need to be addressed to ensure that the woman's care is provided with clinical dexterity include:

- Can I practise this skill in other ways?
- How has my previous experience influenced how I approach this procedure today?
- How can I be sure I am carrying this out correctly?
- Are there opportunities for practising this skill elsewhere?

Models of care

Midwives work in many different settings and in a range of maternity care systems. For example, they may work independently providing holistic client-centred care, or they may work within a large tertiary centre providing care for women with specific health needs. The models of care can be influential in determining the care that a woman may receive, from whom, and when. Midwives need to consider the most appropriate ways that care can be delivered so that they can influence future development in the best interests of women and their families.

Questions that need to be addressed to ensure that the impact of the way that care is provided is acknowledged include:

- How is the maternity service organized?
- Which professional groups are involved in the provision of this service?
- How is this procedure influenced by the model of care provided?
- How does this model of care impact on the carers?
- How does this model of care impact on the woman and her family?

Safe environment

The code of professional conduct states that 'you must act without delay if you believe that you, a colleague or anyone else may be putting someone at risk' (NMC 2008:06). The midwife must ensure that the care she gives does not compromise the safety of women and their families. She must therefore create and maintain a safe working environment at all times, wherever she practises. Questions that need to be addressed to ensure that the woman's care is provided in a safe environment include:

- Are there facilities to ensure that her privacy and dignity are maintained?
- Is there somewhere to wash hands?
- Is there an appropriate place to dispose of waste?

- Is the equipment appropriately maintained and free from contamination?
- Is the space adequate to allow ease of movement around the woman without invading her personal space?
- What are the risks involved in this procedure and how have they been addressed?
- Are there any risks to the person undertaking the procedure?
- Is this environment safe for others who might come into the room?

Promotes health

Providing care for women and their families presents a unique opportunity to influence the health and wellbeing of the public. Midwives must capitalize on their contacts with women to help them achieve a healthy pregnancy and birth and promote lifestyle choices that will benefit women, babies and families in the future. Questions that need to be addressed to ensure that the woman's care promotes health include:

- Is this procedure going to help her or harm her or her baby in any way?

- What are the opportunities to use this procedure to educate her/her family on healthy behaviour?
- What resources can women and families access to help them make healthy lifestyle choices?

The book begins with a chapter focusing on communication. As the jigsaw model shows, effective communication is central to the provision of woman-centred midwifery care. The following chapters then use the jigsaw model to explore scenarios from practice. Thus the reader is provided with a structure with which to reflect on her care and that of the multi-professional team in which she works. Each chapter includes a range of activities designed to enable the midwife to contextualize the information within her own practice, applying her continually developing knowledge to her own circumstances. The chapters are written so that they can be accessed without the previous ones having been read, although we hope you will find the whole book relevant and thought-provoking. Enjoy!

References

Definition of a midwife. Available at: http://www.medicalknowledgeinstitute.com/files/ICM%20Definition%20of%20the%20Midwife%202005.pdf

Department of Health 1993 Changing childbirth: Report of the Expert Maternity Group Pt. II; Report of the Expert Maternity Group Pt. I. Department of Health, London

International Confederation of Midwives Council 2005 Definition of a midwife. Online. Available: http://www.medicalknowledgeinstitute.com/files/

ICM%20definition%20of%20a%20midwife%202005.pdf

Department of Health 2004 Maternity Standard, National Service Framework for children, young people and maternity services. Department of Health, London

Nursing and Midwifery Council (NMC) 2004a Midwives rules and standards. NMC, London

Nursing and Midwifery Council (NMC) 2004b Standards of proficiency for pre registration midwifery education. NMC, London

Nursing and Midwifery Council (NMC) 2007 Introduction of essential skills clusters for pre-registration midwifery education programmes. NMC Circular 23/2007, London

Nursing and Midwifery Council (NMC) 2008 The Code. Standards of conduct, performance and ethics for nurses and midwives. NMC, London.

Wickham S 2004 Feminism and ways of knowing. In: Stewart M (ed) Pregnancy, birth and maternity care: feminist perspectives. Books for Midwives, Oxford, pp 157–168

Chapter 2

Communication

Introduction

The basis of effective caring involves relationship building between the individuals concerned. In order for this relationship to be established appropriate and effective communication must take place. How the woman perceives her carers can make a significant contribution to her evaluation of the birth experience. Women value being cared for by staff who can communicate effectively with them and appreciate the opportunity to get to know their carers (Mackinnon et al 2005). In a study by Kintz (1987) in which women were asked to identify the helpfulness of procedures during labour, it was concluded that, 'interpersonal skills are at least as important as technical skills, if not more so' (p. 30). Also, how professionals communicate with each other has ramifications for how women perceive their care. Such interactions impact on the level of commitment perceived by the woman (Peltier et al 2000). The purpose of this chapter therefore is to highlight the principles of good communication to enable appropriate relationships to be established between the midwife and the families in her care and the multi-professional team.

Trigger scenario

Consider the following scenario in relation to effective communication.

Janine is meeting the midwife Claire for the first time in the antenatal booking clinic. Janine sits with her chin down and stares at the floor. Claire sits at the desk with her side to Janine writing in the notes. 'Everything going ok, Janine?' she asks. 'OK,' Janine mumbles in reply. 'Great,' says Claire. 'Is this your first pregnancy?'

Questions raised by the trigger might include:

- In meeting a person for the first time are there particular ways a midwife should communicate?
- Does the environment make a difference?
- What is Janine communicating by her body language?

- What methods of communication are being used here?
- Is the way the midwife asks questions important?
- What does Janine's response indicate?
- How could Claire have responded differently?

Background

A definition of communication is:

a process that involves a meaningful exchange between at least two people to convey facts, needs, opinions, thoughts, feelings or other information through both verbal and non-verbal means, including face to face exchanges and the written word.

(NHS Modernisation Agency 2003b)

This definition indicates that communication takes place within the context of relationships. It aims to be a 'meaningful exchange' which suggests that it is responsive in some way; its success is dependent on the content of the message, the skills and emotions of the messenger and the context of the recipient's life. There are many aspects of communication and these are now described.

Verbal communication

Verbal communication takes place in a number of different situations. It can be during a face-to-face conversation or by telephone. It may take place on a one-to-one basis, or in a group or lecture setting. It involves the use of words or sounds and language. Verbal communication usually involves two aspects: one person speaking and another listening.

Listening

Listening is a key part of a verbal exchange. Concentrating whilst someone is speaking demonstrates respect for the other person. Not listening carefully can lead to misunderstanding or to the speaker giving up trying to get their message across.

Active listening involves taking time and concentrating on what the other person is trying to convey. It is suggested that three techniques that demonstrate that a person is being listened to include:

- Paraphrasing the speaker's thoughts and feelings
- Expressing understanding of the speaker's feelings
- Asking questions (DeVito 2001).

This process entails 'reflecting back' to the other what has been said to ensure there has been understanding. The application of these skills is also relevant for telephone conversations. The need to speak clearly and listen carefully to what is being said is essential, especially as the cues of body language are not available to assist in interpretation of meaning.

Questioning techniques are relevant to midwifery practice as midwives often need to take a detailed personal history or assess why a woman has presented to the maternity services for care. Questions may be open or closed. Closed questions are generally those to which there is a limited, simple response, for example 'what is your name' or 'where do you live?'. Open questions are those that aim to extract more detail from the person being questioned and give them freedom to express the answer in their own way. Enabling open questions may facilitate the person to provide the information they feel is most relevant for them. This latter form of questioning, although more time-consuming, is essential for the provision of woman-centred care.

Activity

In pairs try one person speaking and the other not paying attention. Note the body language and your feelings during this activity.

Language

It is important to speak in a language that the other person understands. Where the recipient's first language is not English, it may be appropriate to employ the services of a professional interpreter. The use of a client's relations should be avoided for this purpose, except in an emergency, as the individual's culture, age, sex and seniority within a family may influence whether messages are translated verbatum or edited. The client whose first language is not English may be able to understand English very well as long as the midwife speaks clearly and without haste; there is no need to raise one's voice.

How you speak to your family or friends in familiar terms may not be appropriate when talking to clients. Similarly, how professionals speak to each other, using jargon and vernacular, is not appropriate in conversations with women and their families. That is not to say that technical terms cannot be used, but that the midwife should check understanding and offer to interpret some terminology so that women can be involved in their care.

The tone and pitch of voice can also convey emotion. Care should be taken to ensure that one's voice shows interest rather than boredom and concern rather than fear.

Telephone communication

The midwife often communicates with clients or other professionals over the phone. As she does not have the additional information provided by body language she should endeavour to use unambiguous language and a clear voice. She should avoid having three-way conversations, for example if a partner rings in about a woman in labour, as it is difficult to get a true sense of the situation without speaking directly to the woman. Conversations on the phone can lack structure. To ensure that all important information is gathered, for example about a woman in labour or laboratory results, it is useful to have a pro forma or pathway to follow and complete. This should be an aid to care and not applied rigidly in situations where the woman should lead the conversation.

Activity

Access the All Wales clinical pathway for normal labour – telephone advice: http://www.wales.nhs.uk/sites3/Documents/327/Part%20one.pdf

Do you have a similar pro forma where you work?

Currently midwives who work in the community carry mobile phones, radios or pagers. However, on many trust premises and surgeries it is requested that mobile phones are switched off. This may prevent some people being able to communicate with their midwives or with their personal support network. Further work needs to be carried out to establish if the use of mobile phones enables enhanced communication between a midwife and her clients.

Physical communication

Body language

Communication does not just involve the use of words, it includes the use of body posture and gestures to express meaning, a concept also known as 'body language'. A person's facial expression also conveys the emotion behind the words. The use of the hands in the form of gestures or touch also communicates meaning with or without words.

These activities demonstrate how reliant we are on the use of our bodies when we are giving information and the implications for communication when women have restricted movement due to intravenous infusions, pulse oxymetry or intubation.

How we position ourselves during a conversation may also demonstrate how we feel even if our words are contradictory. For example, when we have our arms folded this can convey aggression and hostility, being closed to what the other person is saying. Thus to convey interest and concern the midwife should adopt an open posture, lean forward slightly and maintain eye contact. However, it should be recognized that for people from different cultures the signs of body language may mean different things. The use of gestures and eye contact may be usual practice within our culture but within others their use may be a sign of rudeness or disrespect (Schott & Henley 1996:72, Thompson 2003:29).

Personal space

Recognizing the need for interpersonal space is also a crucial aspect of effective communication. Being too close to a person with whom we are not normally intimate, during a conversation, can make both parties feel uncomfortable. It has been suggested that the usual nose to nose distance during normal social conversation is between 4 and 5 feet (Rungapadiachy 1999) but that different interpersonal distances are appropriate in different situations. As midwives we need to be aware of the impact of our closeness to clients as we are often in a position to be caring for women in very close proximity.

Touch

The way that we touch another individual can express intense meaning to the other. Skill is required to judge whether it is appropriate (Hall 2001). Laying a hand on someone's arm or shoulder can convey concern and caring, but not all women are comfortable with this. Kitzinger (1997) demonstrates the potential for touch to be used as a positive tool for communication or one that can cause emotional distress to the persons concerned. Care should be taken that the other person does not misconstrue the messages that are given through touch. It is therefore advisable to ask permission from the client before using touch in a professional situation and essential prior to intimate examinations.

Activity

Think about how you use touch when communicating. Read Kitzinger (1997). Identify the different forms of touch used in midwifery practice.

Presence

The issue of the presence of the carer in an encounter with those who are being cared for has been suggested to be the ability to be 'in tune' with the other and being aware of the other's uniqueness as a person (Simons 1987).

Different descriptions of 'presence' have been described (Osterman & Schwartz-Barcott, 1996):

■ *Presence* – This is where the carer is physically in the room with another, but totally self-absorbed, and therefore not available to the other.
■ *Partial presence* – This is where the carer is physically present but focuses her energy on a task rather than on the other person.
■ *Full presence* – This is where the carer is physically and psychologically present and each client interaction is 'personalized'.
■ *Transcendent presence* – This is described as 'spiritual' presence and is said to come from a 'spiritual source initiated by centring'. The presence is felt as peaceful, comforting and harmonious. There are seen to be no limits on the role of the carer and that she is able to recognize 'oneness' with the client.

From a midwifery perspective, a study of women's experiences of their midwife showed that the phenomenon of 'presence' is necessary to enable a favourable interaction to occur (Berg et al 1996:15). They suggest that this presence pervades the encounter with the need:

■ To be seen as an individual
■ To have a dependable relationship
■ To have support and be directed on one's own conditions.

The researchers suggested that some midwives were unable to provide this relationship, and were described as 'absently present'. It is clear from this that presence of the participants is required for effective communication to take place.

Activity

Think of those midwives you have worked with. Identify those you consider to have 'presence'? How can you develop this in yourself?

Written communication

Written communication may be used in a number of ways; through letters of introduction, leaflets and information, writing in the maternity record, referral to other professional groups and completion of forms. Professionally it may also include completion of portfolios, reflective activities, essays, articles, completion of records, compilation of reports and statements, completion of charts, or preparing a job application. These activities may need writing in different ways as well as in different mediums. Some will be written by hand while others may require completion through a computer. Whatever ways they are written many are legal documents (Dimond 2004:1159) and therefore care needs to be taken to ensure they are factually correct and do not breach client confidentiality.

Information is often given verbally to women and their families but this should be reinforced where possible through the use of leaflets or information sheets. However, care must be taken as some women may not be able to read or understand the language in which it is written (Smith 2006).

Electronic maternity notes systems have been in place for some time in some areas and a nationwide format is now being developed (Walder 2006). The use of these may change the ways midwives currently document care and enable a more effective strategy, however there may also be anxiety regarding how the data stored will be protected for the wellbeing of the client.

Activity

Think of ways you think that the use of electronic communication may support your practice.

Visual communication

Visual communication may include the use of pictures, such as drawing diagrams to explain issues, the use of graphical representation to replace text, or the use of web based or video material. The use of visual materials is useful to demonstrate situations where women find the verbal explanation difficult or to reinforce what is being said. Examples of visual aids include the use of models in antenatal education or the use of pictures to trigger discussions.

Posters placed on walls in clinics are also visual displays of instructions or health promotion information.

Visual communication may also be established through the woman being encouraged to create pictures herself which the midwife may use as a tool to discuss and explore how the woman is feeling about her pregnancy (England & Horowitz 1998, Hall 2007). Further visual communication may be used to help parents communicate with their unborn baby through the use of cards and activities (Lynch & Bemrose 2005).

To summarize, Box 2.1 lists the factors to be considered when communicating with clients.

Barriers to communication

Communication should be a natural process. However, barriers to its effectiveness can arise, such as:

- Not listening
- Hearing impairment

Box 2.1 Benchmarks of best practice (NHS Modernisation Agency 2003b:02)

Effective interpersonal communication needs to be considered in the context of:

- Fundamental values including openness, honesty and transparency
- The importance of consent and confidentiality
- The principles of common courtesy
- Self-awareness and the importance of body language and other non-verbal communication
- Skills such as establishing rapport, active and empathetic listening, being non-judgemental
- The importance of using straightforward language and avoiding jargon
- The need to adapt approaches to communication, to be sensitive to language and cultural differences (using interpreters where appropriate), to individual developmental needs and disabilities (using aids and appliances as necessary), to the psychological state and the experience of the patient and or carer
- The content of the communication and the situation, such as conveying bad news, dealing with complaints and resolving disputes and hostile situations.

- Use of language that is not understandable, e.g. professional language
- Use of different languages
- Inability to express verbally
- Inability to make eye contact
- Inability to express physically
- Poor use of visual clues
- Impaired telephone contact
- Poor writing skills
- Use of abbreviations that could be misunderstood
- Choice of environment not conducive to appropriate communication
- Fear, anxiety and stress
- Lack of time
- Placing physical barriers between persons, e.g. computers or desks
- Cultural or age differences.

Activity

Consider your own area of work and practice. Looking at the above list, can you identify ways in which you could make changes to reduce the barriers and improve communication?

Within midwifery practice it should also be noted that some women may have more difficulties in communication than others. For example, some women with disabilities such as deafness or forms of aphasia will require special consideration. These may lead to difficulty in expression of her needs as well as understanding. The introduction of the Disability Discrimination Act (2004) has placed responsibility on service providers to consider the needs of those with disabilities which may mean the provision of sign language interpreters and visual displays in clinic areas for those who have hearing difficulties (Panagamuwa et al 2005).

Some mental health conditions will also lead to inability to listen or process the information that is being given. These women may also be affected by the types of treatments or drugs that they are taking. Excessive alcohol intake or recreational drug use may also have an effect on the ability to retain information. Other women who are vulnerable will be those for whom English is not their first language. Schott & Henley (1996) highlight the effect that stress can have, especially in situations where women have a language barrier.

Communication skills

Having established that there are barriers to good communication, midwives need to consider the skills that are required to ensure this is improved. In antenatal care the booking interview is important as it provides the basis from which the rest of the care is planned. One study has demonstrated that different philosophies for communication were used in different models of practice (McCourt 2006). They found that the caseload model of care favoured a less hierarchical and more conversational approach than those employed in conventional care. Women reported that the caseload philosophy afforded them more information, choice and control.

The midwife clearly needs emotional understanding and skills of active listening in order to communicate effectively. She needs to be 'actively present' with the person at that moment in time (Berg et al 1996). She needs to have observation skills and understanding of the visual cues provided by verbal and physical behaviour and to be aware of her own body language. Schott & Henley (1996: 85) suggest ways to reduce stress aimed at women from different cultures, but which could equally be applicable to all women:

- Ensure the woman's name and its pronunciation are correct.
- Allow time or do not show that time is short. Arrange another appointment if necessary.
- Aim to show a sympathetic approach rather than irritation or frustration.
- If the woman is unable to understand verbal communication concentrate on using non-verbal reassurance and behave calmly.
- Observe for signs of the woman and yourself becoming tired by the encounter.
- During procedures keep talking rather than maintaining total silence.
- Aim for continuity of care and maintain notes to prevent repetition from different professionals.
- Aim to learn a few words of the person's language.
- Aim to spend the same amount of time with all women from all cultural backgrounds.

Midwives must recognize the needs of all groups of women, including lesbian women and their partners. One study highlighted how information in waiting areas and leaflets may make assumptions about women's sexuality which can be a barrier to communication (Rondahl et al 2006).

Particular communication skills will be needed to support women with unwell or dying babies or in the presentation of difficult news to members of the family. The 'breaking bad news' website (http://www. breakingbadnews.co.uk/guidelines.asp) provides useful information to health professionals.

Activity

If you have not done so spend some time with another midwife as they give difficult news to a woman and her family. Consider how this was carried out and reflect on how you would handle this situation.

National guidance

Communication between people is a natural part of life. We communicate and respond in the ways that are most effective for us as individuals. However, in professional relationships, the ability to communicate is essential in order to provide the most effective care and meet the needs of the people concerned. Having the skills to develop and maintain these relationships is an important part of midwifery care. Complaints from patients (Commission for Healthcare Audit and Inspection 2006) and reports such as that of the Bristol Inquiry (Kennedy 2001) highlight failures in the systems of care where people had been let down by poor communication. Recognition of this has been highlighted in the NHS Plan (Department of Health 2000) which has led to the development of the Essence of Care Framework as part of the Clinical Governance Strategy for the NHS (NHS Modernisation Agency 2003a). Part of the framework relates to effective communication in which it presents the agreed patient-focused outcome that:

Patients and carers experience effective communication, sensitive to their individual needs and preferences that promotes high quality care for the patient.

(NHS Modernisation Agency 2003b:3)

Box 2.2 Communication: NMC midwifery proficiency (NMC 2004a)

All healthcare personnel demonstrate effective interpersonal skills when communicating with patients and/or carers.

Communication takes place at a time and in an environment that is acceptable to all parties.

All patients' and/or carers' communication needs are assessed on initial contact and are regularly reassessed. Additional communication support is negotiated and provided when a need is identified.

Information that is accessible, acceptable, up to date and meets the needs of individuals is shared actively and consistently with all patients and/or carers and widely promoted across all communities.

Appropriate and effective methods of communication are used actively to promote understanding between patients and/or carers and healthcare personnel.

The principal carer is identified at all times and an assessment is made with them of their needs, involvement, willingness and ability to collaborate with practitioners in order to provide care.

All patients and/or carers are continuously supported and fully enabled to perform their role safely.

All care providers communicate fully and effectively with each other to ensure that patients and/or carers benefit from a comprehensive plan of care which is regularly updated and evaluated.

All patients and/or carers are enabled to communicate their individual needs and preferences at all times.

Effective communication ensures and demonstrates that the patients' and/or carers' expert contribution to care is valued, recorded, reviewed and informs both patient care and healthcare personnel education.

All the patients' and/or carers' information, support and training needs are jointly identified, agreed, met and regularly reviewed.

To aid the achievement of this outcome, benchmarks of best practice have been developed to enable practitioners to create services that will facilitate this process (Box 2.2).

The importance of effective communication is raised in the *National Service Framework for children, young people and maternity services* (Department of Health 2004:08). It states that women should be given clear information on the choices available to them and:

... enough time between receiving information and making choices to reflect upon the information, consider their options and seek additional information and advice where they wish to.

This places the onus on the professionals caring for a woman to give her the options she needs in a language that she understands. The framework continues by stating that women should be given a copy of their care pathway with an explanation to enable them to access further services if required. The care pathway must therefore be created and written in such a way that all women will be able to understand its meaning. The needs of women from cultural groups where English is not their first language are also discussed within the document alongside those women who may have learning or physical disabilities. Provision of support through translation or interpreting services is encouraged along with assessing ways services can be changed to increase access by these groups.

The intrapartum care guidelines (NICE 2007:17) have a dedicated section describing how healthcare professionals should establish communication with the labouring woman, and many are transferable to the care of women who access maternity services at any time. Of particular importance is 'maintain a calm and confident approach so that their demeanour reassures the woman that all is going well'. It reminds professionals to be self-aware and consider the impact of body language and behaviour on the women in their care.

Postnatal care is highlighted in the NSF (Department of Health 2004) as a time when women tend to receive conflicting advice and the need to establish appropriate care plans is recommended for this time. The provision of health promotion information for parents is also raised as an issue. The NSF (Department of Health 2004) clearly documents that good communication is necessary in the maternity services to facilitate the best care.

Ensuring good communication channels are in place to provide appropriate information and explanations will help enable women to have confidence in their carers, to build up trusting relationships with a known, named midwife, to have personalized care and feel safe in their environment.

Professional regulation

Midwives who work in the United Kingdom must work within the regulatory framework of the Nursing and Midwifery Council. Their code of professional conduct (NMC 2008:05) requires all registrants to:

... work cooperatively within teams and respect the skills, expertise and contributions of your colleagues.

Activity

List the different professionals that are involved in maternity care. Find out what systems are in place where you work to foster interprofessional communication

For midwives the expectation is that communication skills will be learnt through education programmes, ensuring students are able to communicate effectively with women and their families and other members of the healthcare team in order to provide appropriate woman-centred care. In addition students should receive training on information giving and the completion of maternity records (NMC 2004). In order to fulfil professional requirements the student midwife must demonstrate competence in all 29 midwifery proficiencies described in Standard 15. Sections of Standard 15 that have relevance to communication skills are laid out in Box 2.3:

Box 2.3 Effective midwifery practice (NMC 2004:09)

Effective midwifery practice will be demonstrated by being able to:

1. Communicate effectively with women and their families throughout the pre-conception, antenatal, intrapartum and postnatal periods.

   Communication will include:

   - listening to women, jointly identifying their feelings and anxieties about their pregnancies, the birth and the related changes to themselves and their lives
   - enabling women to think through their feelings
   - enabling women to make informed choices about their health and healthcare
   - actively encouraging women to think about their own health and the health of their babies and families, and how this can be improved
   - communicating with women throughout their pregnancy, labour and the period following birth.

2. Care for, monitor and support women during labour and monitor the condition of the fetus and support spontaneous births. This will include:

   - communicating with women throughout and supporting them through the experience.

3. Complete, store and retain records of practice which:

   - are accurate, legible and continuous
   - detail the reasoning behind any actions taken
   - contain the information necessary for the record's purpose.

   Records will include:

   - biographical details of women and babies' assessments made, outcomes of assessments and the action taken as a result
   - the outcomes of discussions with women and the advice offered
   - any drugs administered
   - action plans and commentary on their evaluation.

Activity

Access the full document and look at the whole of Standard 15 (NMC 2004). Apply these to your current experience of practice. Observe other midwives and consider how they are communicating. How can you demonstrate progress towards competence with regard to communication?

Reflection on trigger scenario

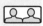

Janine is meeting the midwife Claire for the first time in the antenatal booking clinic. Janine sits with her chin down and stares at the floor. Claire sits at the desk with her side to Janine writing in the notes. 'Everything going ok, Janine?' she asks. 'OK,' Janine mumbles in reply. 'Great,' says Claire. 'Is this your first pregnancy?'

This scenario highlights a situation where the midwife could have behaved differently to ensure effective communication with Janine, whom she was meeting for the first time. Claire should have been prepared for meeting Janine and welcomed her appropriately. It is clear that the environment is not conducive to the asking of sensitive questions. Claire could have ensured the layout of the room had been changed so that she was not sitting at the desk and was in a position to write and talk to Janine and face her at the same time. Further, she may have considered asking Janine if she would like the booking interview to be carried out within Janine's home environment as this may promote Janine's comfort and may enable Claire to find out more about her.

The way that she asked the question is also relevant. She chose to use a closed question and so Janine gave a monosyllabic answer. Using open questions in this situation and offering Janine an open body and eye contact may have encouraged Janine to reveal more of her concerns. If she had been looking at Janine when her answers were given she may have established from the body language and the tone of language used that the answers Janine gave had not revealed the whole truth of what she was feeling. Claire's reply also demonstrates a poor response to Janine's answer and thus closes off the opportunity to continue the conversation.

Further scenarios

The following scenarios enable you to consider how specific situations influence the care a midwife provides. Consider the following in relation to the principles of effective communication.

Scenario 1

Hannah is planning to lead an antenatal education session focusing on postnatal issues. She is aware that 15 couples will be attending and she wants to try and include everyone in the discussion.

Practice point

Providing preparation for childbirth workshops in a way that meets the needs of the whole group presents a challenge for midwives. Each individual will come to the group with a range of expectations and previous life experiences that will impact on their information needs. The midwife must not only take into account the need to facilitate effective communication between herself and the group but also encourage members of the group to interact with each other so that they can share insights and experiences.

Questions

Has Hannah undertaken a similar session before?
What educational preparation has Hannah had to enable her to lead such a group?
Where is the session taking place, at what time and for how long?
What might be the barriers to effectively communicating the issues to the group?
What techniques could Hannah use to ensure everyone is involved in the session?

Scenario 2

Eleanor is on duty on the postnatal ward. She goes to answer a call bell from a side ward. 'What can I do for you?' she asks as she enters. The woman in the bed, Julie, does not answer her. Instead she points to her hearing aid in her hand that is clearly not working for her.

Practice point

Midwives care for women with a range of communication needs. Each woman's individual circumstances need to be assessed and regularly evaluated to ensure that the care they receive continues to meet their specific requirements.

- What assessments have been made of Julie's communication needs?
- Does Julie have a named midwife caring for her?
- Who else could help facilitate effective communication with Eleanor and her carers?
- What could Eleanor have found out before she entered the room?
- Consider how Eleanor will now communicate with Julie.
- What resources are available to enable midwives to meet the needs of deaf women in their care?

Conclusion

This chapter has highlighted why midwives need to develop communication skills for the benefit of the women and families in their care. It has described the different forms of communication and the ways they can be used in midwifery practice. It is recognized that the best forms of communication occur when a relationship has been established, therefore midwives should consider ways they could improve the organization of maternity care to enhance the development of relationships and facilitate the most effective means of communication.

Useful resources

All Wales clinical pathway for normal labour – telephone advice
http://www.wales.nhs.uk/sites3/Documents/327/Part%20one.pdf

Intrapartum care guideline NICE clinical guideline 55
http://guidance.nice.org.uk/CG55

Essence of care programme
http://www.cgsupport.nhs.uk/Programmes/Essence_of_Care_Programme/

References

Berg M, Lundgren I, Lindmark G 2005 A midwifery model of care for childbearing women at high risk: genuine caring in caring for the genuine. Journal of Perinatal Education 14(1): 9–21

Commission for Healthcare Audit and Inspection 2006 State of healthcare 2006. Commision for Healthcare, London

Department of Health 2000 The NHS Plan: a plan for investment, a plan for reform. Department of Health, London

Department of Health 2004 Maternity Standard, National Service Framework for children, young people and maternity services. Department of Health, London

Devito J A 2001 Essentials of human communication, 4th edn. Addison-Wesley, Harlow

Dimond B 2004 Law and the midwife. In: Henderson C, MacDonald S (eds) Mayes' midwifery: a textbook for midwives. Baillière Tindall, Oxford

Disability Discrimination Act 2004. HMSO, London

England P, Horowitz R 1998 Birthing from within. Partera Press, Albuquerque

Hall J 2001 Midwifery mind and spirit: emerging issues of care. Books for midwives, Oxford

Hall J 2007 Creativity, spirituality and birth. In: Davis L (ed) Art and soul of birth. Books for midwives, Oxford

Kennedy I 2001 Learning from Bristol: the Report of the public inquiry into children's heart surgery at the Bristol Royal Infirmary 1984–1995. Department of Health, London

Kintz D 1987 Nursing support in labour. Journal of Obstetric, Gynecologic and Neonatal Nursing 16(2): 126–130

Kitzinger S 1997 Authoritative touch in childbirth – a cross-cultural approach. In: Davis Floyd R E, Sargent C F (eds) Childbirth and authoritative knowledge: cross-cultural perspectives. University of California Press, Berkeley

Lynch L, Bemrose S 2005 It's good to talk: pre- and post-birth interaction. Practising Midwife 8(3): 17–20

McCourt C 2006 Supporting choice and control? Communication and interaction between midwives and women at the antenatal booking visit. Social Science and Medicine 62: 1307–1318

MacKinnon K, McIntyre M, Quance M 2005 The meaning of the nurse's presence during childbirth. Journal of Obstetric, Gynecologic and Neonatal Nursing 34(1): 28–36

NHS Modernisation Agency 2003a Essence of care: patient-focused benchmarks for clinical governance. Department of Health, London. Online. Available: http://www.cgsupport.nhs.uk/Programmes/Essence_of_Care_Programme/The_Ten_Benchmarks.asp# 17 Oct 2006

NHS Modernisation Agency 2003b Benchmarks for communication between patients, carers and health care personnel. Department of Health, London. Online. Available: http://www.cgsupport.nhs.uk/downloads/Essence_of_Care/Communication.doc Accessed: 17/10/06

National Institute for Health and Clinical Excellence (NICE) 2007 Intrapartum care. Care of healthy women and their babies during childbirth. NICE clinical guideline 55. NICE, London

Nursing and Midwifery Council (NMC) 2004 Standards of proficiency for pre-registration midwifery education. NMC, London

Nursing and Midwifery Council (NMC) 2008 The Code. Standards of conduct, performance and ethics for nurses and midwives. NMC, London

Osterman P, Schwartz-Barcott 1996 Presence: four ways of being there. Nursing Forum 31(2): 23–30

Panagamuwa C, Wellman K, Davidson M 2005 Communicating with deaf patients. BMJ Careers 330: 7494

Peltier J, Schibrowski J, Westfall J 2000 Exploring the role nurses play at different stages of the birthing process. Marketing Health Services Fall: 21–28

Rondahl G, Innala S, Carlsson M 2006 Heterosexual assumptions in verbal and non-verbal communication in nursing. Journal of Advanced Nursing 56(4): 373–381

Rungapadiachy D 1999 Interpersonal communication and psychology for health care professionals. Butterworth Heinemann, Oxford

Schott J, Henley A 1996 Culture and religion and childbearing in a multiracial society: a handbook for health professionals. Butterworth Heinemann, Oxford

Simons J 1987 Patients' and nurses' perception of caring. The research review: practice studies for nursing 4: 2

Smith S 2006 Cross cultural information leaflets. Nursing Standard 21(4): 39–41

Thompson N 2003 Communication and language: a handbook of theory and practice. Palgrave Macmillan, London

Walder J 2006 A vision of the future. RCM Midwives 9(2): 64–65

Chapter 3

Hygiene and infection control: the immobile woman

Introduction

Being able to move around and attend to our own hygiene needs are activities that we often take for granted. Most of us have the choice about whether we want to wash, shower or have a bath on a regular basis without considering whether we can physically use the facilities that are available. We do not think about sitting or lying in a bed or chair for a long time without being able to move or the implications this may have on our bodies. Similarly, fit and healthy pregnant women may not consider the potential impact of an epidural or operative birth on their mobility and independence. Rising caesarean section and epidural rates (The Information Centre 2006) as well as increasing rates of obesity (Zaninotto et al 2006) mean that midwives require knowledge and understanding of how immobility may impact on women's care needs. In addition, increasing numbers of women with reduced mobility are having babies. Thus some women will require assistance to maintain their personal cleanliness.

The aim of this chapter is to highlight the skills required by midwives to care for women who are immobile or in bed for a period of time. These include attending to women's personal hygiene needs, maintaining skin integrity through appropriate pressure area care and taking action to reduce the introduction and spread of infection.

Trigger scenario

In the following scenario consider hygiene, mobility and infection control issues:

Samantha has given birth to Jessica, her first baby, at home. It has been a long labour for her and she is seated on the floor of the sitting room. 'I don't think I can make it into the bath,' she says. It is clear she is splashed with meconium and blood. 'Don't worry, if you would like I will give you a bed bath,' says Marion, the midwife.

The following questions may come to mind:

- Why would it be appropriate to clear the splashes of meconium and blood from Samantha's body?

- What is a bed bath?
- Why did Marion choose to give a bed bath instead of putting Samantha in the bath?
- What equipment is needed to carry out a bed bath?
- How does the environment impact on Samantha's mobility and hygiene needs?
- What other issues may need to be considered if Samantha stays in bed for a long time?

Skin integrity

Background physiology

The skin is the largest organ of the body. One of its many functions, along with the underlying tissue, is to act as a protective barrier to the rest of the body. It protects from impact, such as falls, from heat and cold and external contaminants such as bacteria. The skin also acts as a temperature control regulator, ensuring we are not too hot or too cold, and helps to excrete waste matter. It also has an important sensory function as well as synthesising vitamin D from sunlight.

Activity

Revise the anatomy and normal functions of the skin. Consider a time when the integrity of your skin was compromised: what contributed to this and how was it resolved?

Healthy skin requires adequate amounts of water and a balanced diet in order to function correctly. Underlying health conditions may have an effect on the skin functioning, for example,

anaemia or thyroid conditions may lead to excessive dryness. Further issues such as poor diet or obesity may have an effect on the skin's elasticity or integrity.

Activity

Investigate what effect obesity or anaemia will have on the skin.

Physiology in relation to pregnancy

In a healthy non-pregnant situation the skin will be affected by the inner health and wellbeing of the person as indicated above. However, during pregnancy, the changes happening to the rest of the body will also have an effect on the integrity and functioning of the skin. The extra weight that the body carries, the circulating pregnancy hormones and the needs of the growing fetus will have an effect on all tissues within the body. Conditions that cause intense irritation of the skin may also lead the woman to scratch and break the integrity of the skin, leading to inflammation, pain and potential sites of infection.

Activity

Name the hormones that circulate in pregnancy. Consider the effects of these hormones on the skin. List four conditions that cause itching in pregnancy.

The process of labour also challenges the skin's capacity to fulfil its role. For example, the exertion of labour will increase the body's heat production.

The skin has an important function in maintaining an optimum body temperature. Flushing of the skin, due to vasodilation of the blood vessels beneath the skin's surface, facilitates the loss of heat from the blood. Increased sweat production also aids heat loss through evaporation. It is important therefore that the woman remains well hydrated during labour and as mobile as possible.

Pressure area care

Potential damage to skin may occur in situations where women are immobile or have sensory loss, for example following administration of an epidural or postoperatively. Prolonged pressure on the tissues results in occlusion of the capillaries leading to a build-up of waste products and deprivation of oxygen in the tissues. This pressure, if not relieved, can result in tissue discoloration and damage and in the development of pressure ulcers. These are defined as:

identified damage to an individual's skin due to the effects of pressure together with, or independently from a number of other factors for example shearing, friction and moisture

(NHS Modernisation Agency 2003c:1)

Such ulcers are also be known as 'decubitus ulcers', 'bed sores' or 'pressure sores'. The care employed to prevent them is known as 'pressure area care'.

Local risk factors:

- Pressure
- Capillary occlusion and disruption of lymphatic drainage
- Shearing force
- Increased temperature and moisture.

Systemic risk factors:

- Ageing
- Decreased mobility
- Poor nutrition
- Arterial disease and hypotension.

Women in labour may have many of these risk factors. Pressure can also be increased due to creases in bed linen and skin integrity compromised by contamination with fluids such as liquor or blood. Thus bed linen and clothing should be regularly inspected for creases and kept clean and dry. Further, there should be awareness of labouring women who spend lengths of time in the hands and knees position and whether the surfaces are suitable to support her appropriately. The increased levels of cortisol in labour may also potentially lead to a greater risk of pressure damage to the skin. During labour there should be adequate preparation to ensure the most appropriate equipment is available to aid mobility and that staff know how to use it.

Activity

Identify six areas of the body at risk of pressure damage due to immobility.

Vohra & McCollum (1994) summarize the risk factors for damage to pressure areas as follows.

Activity

Sit on a chair or in a bed for as long as you can without moving. How long did it take before you felt you had to move to get comfortable? Try this also kneeling on the floor or bed. Apply this to midwifery practice.

Assessment of pressure areas

Staying in one position for even a short time may lead to increased pressure on the area in contact with the bed or the floor and may cause skin damage. The risk is exacerbated for women who have underlying medical disorders affecting the elasticity and tone of the skin. In addition, women who have anaemia, poor nutritional status or have some form of disability that prevents mobility or skin sensation have an increased risk of ulcer formation.

To ensure appropriate assessment is made of pressure areas it is suggested a scoring system is used which enables recognition of those who are most at risk of skin damage. The most usual ones to be used are the Waterlow (2005) score and the Plymouth assessment scale, specifically for maternity pressure areas (Morison & Baker 2001). This latter scale enables the midwife to consider the needs of the woman in an holistic way; however, scales need to be used regularly as the woman's condition changes and they should be regarded as risk assessment tools.

Pressure area care aims to protect the areas of the body in contact with the bed or floor and to maintain mobility where women are unable to do so themselves. This will involve regularly changing the person's position but also considering ways of ensuring comfort on the surface on which they may be sitting, lying or leaning. This will include considering the type of mattress used, whether sheets are smooth and dry, and whether floor surfaces require carpets or cushions to aid comfort.

Hygiene

Midwives need to take note of their own personal hygiene and the cleanliness of the working environment, to avoid the transfer of infection to mothers and babies. A focus on clinical hygiene has become acute in recent years with the increased prevalence of 'superbugs' such as methicillin resistant *Staphlococcus Aureus* (MRSA) and *Clostridium difficile*, which remain difficult to treat and can have a devastating effect on those who contract them (Crowcroft & Catchpole 2002). This has led to an increased emphasis on techniques to contain or prevent infection and raised expectations of those accessing health services for scrupulous hygiene standards. Simple techniques such as careful handwashing and appropriate disposal of waste can significantly reduce the transmission of infection. It is ironic that our current understanding of cross infection developed through the observations of a Hungarian obstetrician, Ignaz Semmelweis, who in 1847 recognized that the spread of puerperal infection in hospital in Vienna was through the poor hygiene of medical students (Rotter 1998).

Carers should use appropriate handwashing techniques to prevent cross infection to either the mother or the infant. The newborn infant has a less efficient immune system than an adult and is therefore at greater risk of

Activity

Access the poster at http://www.hse.gov.uk/skin/posters/skinwashing.pdf and learn how to wash your hands appropriately.

Consider your workplace and whether the facilities are available to ensure appropriate hygiene.

contracting infection. If in hospital it may be wise to minimize contact with the infant from others apart from the parents and ensure careful handwashing.

Asepsis is defined as 'the prevention of microbial contamination of living tissue/fluid or sterile materials by excluding, removing or killing micro-organsims' (Xavier 1999). The aim of this is to prevent infection. The different ways this can be done is by:

- The use of antiseptic solutions as a preventative measure
- Cleaning to remove dirt
- Disinfection to remove micro-organisms
- Sterilization to completely remove all micro-organisms and bacterial spores.

(Xavier 1999)

Activity

Think about the above list and apply this to your current practice area. Which activities that you have seen use these methods to prevent infection?

The later chapter on surgical care will consider the actual techniques used in asepsis for wounds. However, midwives may consider when the use of an aseptic technique may be required for other procedures such as catheterization of a woman or vaginal examination (Stewart 2005). For each type of procedure different gloves will be recommended according to the area in which you are working.

National guidance

Recognition of patient care needs has led to the development of the Essence of Care Framework as part of the Clinical

Activity

Find out in your area of work which gloves are recommended for the following:

- A non-sterile contact with a woman
- Aseptic technique
- Vaginal examination prior to membranes being ruptured
- Vaginal examination after the membranes have been ruptured
- Administration of suppositories
- Cleaning equipment.

Governance Strategy for the NHS (NHS Modernisation Agency 2003a). This has included benchmarks to be achieved for personal and oral hygiene.

Activity

Consider Benchmarks for Personal and Oral Hygiene (NHS Modernisation Agency 2003b) by accessing the complete document at http://www.cgsupport.nhs.uk/downloads/Essence_of_Care/Personal_&_Oral_Hygiene.doc. How would you apply the information to midwifery practice?

The basic principles forming this document highlight that personal hygiene should be taken seriously for all women in the maternity services. Hygiene is also a significant issue in relation to the prevention of infection to the woman, her baby and also to the midwives and other people caring for them. As indicated in the introduction, infection control has become a major concern especially within hospitals (Crowcroft & Catchpole 2002, Healthcare Commission 2006). This has led to an increased focus on preventative measures for the protection of all. From a maternity service perspective the National Service Framework highlights the need to address poor standards of hygiene, particularly in relation to the postnatal period (Department of Health 2004).

In 2004 the National Patient Safety Agency introduced the 'cleanyourhands' campaign to encourage staff to adhere to more rigid handwashing techniques with 'it's ok to ask' 'policing' by the client to ensure staff followed these principles (National Patient Safety Agency (NPSA) 2004). The NPSA in 2005 instructed the NHS to provide an alcohol handrub near the patient and to encourage its use.

Activity

In your place of work find all the places where handrubs are situated and read any notices nearby. Who are these aimed at and why?

Recognition of the need to reduce infection rates within the health services has led to a Code of Practice to prevent infections related to healthcare (Department of Health 2006). Managing structures of the NHS have responsibilities to those who are admitted to the premises as service users as well as to the members of staff who work there. Their responsibilities lie in a duty to have management systems and training in place to ensure the protection of everyone who enters hospitals from hospital acquired infection (HAI). They have

responsibilities for cleanliness and isolation facilities and information. Uniform, handwashing, cleaning services and waste disposal are policies that are created to ensure that staff and patients are protected by the management guidelines.

Activity

Find out what training and information is provided for staff working in the area where you are located.

Essence of care also has benchmarks in relation to mobility and the protection of the person's skin while their mobility is reduced (NHS Modernisation Agency 2003c).

Activity

Consider the benchmarks for pressure ulcers by accessing the complete document at www.cgsupport.nhs. uk/downloads/Essence_of_Care/ Pressure_Ulcers.doc How would you apply the information to midwifery practice?

Professional regulation

Midwives working within the NHS have a responsibility to abide by the directives of the Trust in which they work. However, the Professional Code of Conduct also applies for the responsibilities and duty you have towards the women and families in your care which would include any midwife practising in or out of the NHS (NMC 2008:06):

"you must report your concerns in writing if problems in the environment of care are putting people at risk."

Standards of education require students to be giving care that is appropriate to the needs of the individual woman from the antenatal period through labour and birth and in the postnatal period (NMC 2004). Midwives should be trained to promote the health and wellbeing of the woman and her baby and specifically:

Care for and monitor women during the puerperium, offering the necessary evidence-based advice and support regarding the baby and self-care. This will include: providing advice and support on feeding babies and teaching women about the importance of nutrition in child development, providing advice and support on hygiene, safety, protection, security and child development.

(NMC 2004:40-1)

NMC (2005) infection control advice includes the standard precautions staff should apply when caring for patients to reduce infection rates:

- Maintain hand hygiene
- Use protective equipment
- Dispose of and use sharps safely
- Dispose of clinical waste safely
- Manage blood and body fluids safely
- Decontaminate equipment appropriately
- Maintain cleanliness of the general environment.

Equipment required to provide hygiene and mobility care

In order to provide appropriate hygienic care for women who are unable to do so for themselves, knowledge will be required on washing in bed and pressure area care. Basic equipment that will be required will be a plastic wash bowl, hand hot water, toiletries (usually the woman's own), towels, mouthwash or toothpaste and toothbrush, clean linen, linen skip, rubbish bag, clean nightwear, apron, non-sterile gloves, sanitary towels, hairbrush, and a cup of clean water and syringe (if the woman is unconscious). Research into nursing students' first bathing experience of patients demonstrated that they felt anxiety (Wolf 1997). They were most uncomfortable about exposing and touching the body parts of another and were surprised by the way that patients helped them through the bath.

Activity

Consider how you feel or felt about carrying out your first bed bath. Put yourself in the woman's position and think how she may be feeling. How do you think you can/could make the experience better for both of you?

Procedure for giving a bed bath

1. The midwife discusses the procedure with the woman, enabling her to understand its relevance to her care and give her consent

Consideration of a woman-centred approach to immobility and hygiene is vital. Women are individual and the importance and significance they apply to personal cleanliness will be personal. Therefore the woman should be central to the development of the plan of care, her views and opinions should be identified and addressed to ensure her needs are met. The midwife

---

Box 3.1   Procedure for giving a bed bath

- **Explain carefully to the woman what you are intending to do**
  Rationale To ensure she is aware of what this entails and can give her consent

- **Ensure that she has had adequate pain relief if required and that this is effective**
  Rationale To ensure that she is not experiencing discomfort during the procedure

- **Obtain all equipment that will be required**
  Rationale To ensure that you will not have to leave her uncovered during the procedure to get equipment

- **Place clean equipment away from the dirty skip and linen**
  Rationale To prevent contamination of the clean equipment

- **Assess her ability to move and get manual handling tools or another person as required**
  Rationale To ensure manual handling requirements are met and ensure protection of yourself and the woman

- **Shut any windows and turn off fans**
  Rationale To ensure the area remains warm during exposure

- **Close curtains around the bed or ensure window blinds are closed in single rooms**
  Rationale To ensure privacy and preserve dignity

- **Put on a plastic apron and wash hands carefully**
  Rationale To protect your uniform from getting wet and to protect the woman from cross infection from anything you are carrying on your uniform or on your hands

- **Tell the woman what you are about to do during the procedure and ensure she gives consent**
  Rationale To ensure that she has adequate information and may refuse if she wishes

- **Remove the bedclothes expect for a top sheet, and ask her to remove her nightwear, if she is able, or assist her**
  Rationale To preserve her dignity as much as possible

- **Ask what she usually uses to wash her face**
  Rationale To ensure you use her normal toiletries and involve her in her care

- **Cover the top half of her chest with a towel and ask her to wash and dry her face, or help her do it**
  Rationale To prevent water dripping onto her chest and to encourage her to move if she is able

- **Exposing the arm furthest away from you, wash this and the armpit, and then dry. Repeat with her chest and neck and then the arm closest to you**
  Rationale To ensure minimal exposure and to keep the woman as warm as possible

- **Carefully wash under the breasts and dry well**
  Rationale To remove any sweat or moisture that may encourage the build-up of micro-organisms

- **Cover the chest area and place the leg furthest away from you on a towel. Wash and dry this and then repeat with the leg closest to you**
  Rationale To prevent excess water from dripping onto the bedclothes

continued

Box 3.1 continued

- Ask the woman to sit forward in bed and place the towel behind her or turn her on her side away from you with her back facing you, well supported, or with an assistant present
  Rationale To expose her back for washing and ensure she does not fall off the bed

- Place a towel behind her and wash and dry her back
  Rationale To prevent excess water from dripping onto the bedclothes

- Establish if she is able to wash her own perineal area through supported sitting on a bedpan or if she requires you to do this
  Rationale To preserve her dignity as much as possible

- If the woman is on a bedpan, ask the assistant to support her and provide warm water in a jug for her to pour over her genital area. Provide disposable wipes as required to dry the area and dispose of in the bedpan
  Rationale To ensure she does not fall off. To prevent contamination of the face flannel

- If the woman is on her side, put on disposable gloves and wash the area with disposable wipes from the vulva towards the buttocks, disposing into a waste bag
  Rationale To prevent contamination of the urethral and vaginal areas with faeces or external skin organisms and to ensure waste is disposed of correctly

- Give the woman a clean sanitary pad or apply one over her perineal area
  Rationale To protect this now clean area when turning her and as some

blood pooled in the vagina may also leak on movement

- Remove the gloves and dispose of them (unless the sheets are very soiled and require changing)
  Rationale To ensure no contamination of clean areas takes place

- Consider which bedding needs changing and assess the woman's ability to get out and sit by the bed while this takes place. Replace nightwear at this time if required and use any toiletries she may wish
  Rationale To ensure that women who are ill are not disturbed unnecessarily. It may be less stressful to encourage the woman to sit out rather than try and change the sheets under her

- Change any sheets as required by rolling her, lifting her or mobilizing her onto a chair and dispose of dirty linen in the appropriate linen skip
  Rationale To ensure the woman is comfortable in bed and ensure no cross infection takes place through the use of the wrong bags

- Assist the woman into a comfortable position back in bed or on the chair
  Rationale To ensure that her needs are met

- Wash and dry your hands
  Rationale To ensure no contamination takes place

- Support her in cleaning her teeth or carry out oral hygiene – use the woman's toothbrush if possible and the syringe and water to aid in rinsing. Assess the condition of her mouth and lips
  Rationale To ensure that her mouth is kept clean and to promote wellbeing. To observe if there are any signs of

continued

Box 3.1 continued

infection or poor health and to prevent dryness

- **Assist her in brushing her hair or do it for her**
  Rationale To promote psychological wellbeing
- **Carry out any further assessment procedures required**

Rationale To ensure there is limited disruption to the woman

- **Document any observations you have made**
  Rationale To ensure the appropriate information is passed on to other colleagues and to prevent repetition of procedures.

should explain everything that will take place and obtain consent for this intimate activity. For women who have partners or other members of the family present, especially within a home environment, respect should also be given to the woman's wishes about their involvement in her care. It is also important to give specific consideration to women who are used to having carers take care of their hygiene needs, because of disability for example, as they may favour a particular routine. If the woman is unconscious clear communication of the procedure should be continued as her hearing may still be intact and she should be kept informed of what you are doing.

Activity

Consider how you would explain to a woman the need for care of her personal hygiene following the birth of her baby. If you can, practise through role-play with a partner.

We need to recognize the psychological impact of remaining immobile for any length of time. The expectation is that women will have a normal, physiological experience of birth and will expect to be well. If they are not expecting an epidural or caesarean section they may feel shocked and distressed by their inability to move or care for themselves. They may feel pain but also embarrassment at needing someone else to care for them. In pregnancy and during labour they may have experienced feeling very hot and sweaty. They may have become splashed or even covered in large amounts of liquor, meconium, blood, urine, faeces or vomit. Not only will this be unpleasant but there may also be cultural, religious or personal reasons as to why they feel upset by this and feel 'unclean'.

Women may also have difficulty in allowing someone who is not intimately associated with them to touch them and the midwife will need sensitivity to assess who the best person may be to provide any hygiene care that is required. It may be appropriate to ask the woman to do as much as she can for herself and possibly ask the partner or her mother to be involved in the care as well. A woman may also feel great embarrassment at exposing her naked body to another and minimal exposure, sensitivity and privacy should be paramount in carrying out any procedures.

2. The procedure is carried out at the appropriate time according to the woman's plan of care

Ideally this should be carried out prior to her eating a meal. It should be ensured that adequate pain relief has been given and is effective before carrying out procedures that may require movement and it should be ensured that communication is with the woman and not over her to another colleague who may be present. If possible the woman's own toiletries should be used in the way she would use them herself. The basic reason for the bed bath is cleanliness for the woman; however it is also an opportunity for assessment of her total wellbeing. Any other examinations or procedures that need to be carried out may all be carried out at the same time. The equipment that is required will depend on the individual needs of the woman and her condition at the time. Planning should mean that the midwife will not need to leave the woman's bedside unnecessarily. This will prevent unnecessary disruption and discomfort for the woman at a later time and will also save time for the midwife.

It is therefore appropriate to plan the procedure carefully at a time when the midwife can give full attention to the woman and with minimum disruption by other members of the multidisciplinary team. The bed bath also offers the opportunity to communicate with the woman deeply and assess her needs. Appropriate care planning and documentation is key to ensuring the woman's needs are met. Attending to the hygiene needs of a woman who is unable to care for herself is a significant part of a midwife's role, as this helps maintain the woman's self-esteem and protects her from infection. Other carers who could be involved are maternity care assistants who may be given guidance to provide a bed bath, change a bed or move the woman as required to ensure pressure area care is given. With women who are totally immobile two members of the team will be required to ensure protection for the woman and the helpers when handling her. Team working with those who clean the ward areas will also ensure that cleaning is carried out at a different time from bathing. Effective communication with other members of the team will also ensure privacy for a woman who may be exposed during a bed bath.

3. The procedure is carried out using the correct technique

The procedure for carrying out a bed bath is explained in Box 3.1. Skewes (1996) writes of the need to carry out bathing in an appropriate way:

- Decide whether it is necessary to bathe at all as it can dry the skin and lead to a greater chance of skin breakdown.
- Use liquid, non-antimicrobial soap, neutral in pH and containing moisturizers.
- Clean washing basins thoroughly between patients.
- Avoid using oils that remain in the bath.

4. The woman is supported during the procedure and her reaction observed

Women who usually require bed baths are generally not well enough to care for themselves, therefore it is essential to carry this out with gentleness and awareness of any reactions that the woman may have. She should be closely observed for signs of pain and level of consciousness.

Observation and assessment of the woman's skin integrity may be carried out during a bed bath. This is of particular importance if she has been immobile for any length of time.

5. The woman is made comfortable after the procedure

Following a bed bath the woman should be left in a comfortable position with a hand bell accessible for her to call for assistance. The sheets should be straight and comfortable and she should be covered to ensure her dignity is preserved before any curtains or doors are opened. Any drinks or food should be placed where she can reach them if required.

6. The woman is informed of the result

If observation of her skin reveals the presence of damage the woman should be informed and encouraged to move regularly if she is able. If she is unconscious carers should return regularly to ensure vulnerable pressure points are relieved and assessed.

7. If the result is outside normal parameters it is reported to an appropriate member of the team

If the bed bath demonstrates that the woman is in excessive pain, is

haemorrhaging or has damaged skin, or any other observations are outside normal parameters, these should be reported to the appropriate member of the team. Support with advice regarding the management and care of women with skin damage may also be obtained from tissue specialist nurses.

8. An accurate and legible record is made of the observation

Recording that the procedure has been completed in the notes will ensure that there will be no wasted time for other members of the team. Any concerns regarding pressure areas should be recorded clearly to identify the need for caution to other members of the team.

Reflection on trigger scenario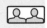

Consider the trigger scenario at the start of the chapter:

Samantha has given birth to Jessica, her first baby, at home. It has been a long labour for her and she is seated on the floor of the sitting room. 'I don't think I can make it into the bath,' she says. It is clear she is splashed with meconium and blood. 'Don't worry, if you would like I will give you a bed bath,' says Marion, the midwife.

The scenario involves a woman following birth, although the issues that have been raised above could be applied to any situation where a woman becomes immobile either during pregnancy or beyond. This chapter has explored the physiological and psychological issues around caring for women in this situation and you will have more insight into the issues in the scenario. The jigsaw model will be used to consider the issues in more depth.

Effective communication

In all aspects of maternity care it is important to communicate appropriately and effectively. When dealing with personal issues, such as hygiene and mobility, sensitivity is important in the way that communication takes place. Women may get the impression that midwives are in a hurry which may lead to women feeling reluctant to ask for assistance in caring for their everyday needs. From this scenario we could ask: Have Samantha and Marion built a trusting relationship in pregnancy already? Has Marion already started running a bath, assuming this will be what Samantha wants to do? Has she asked Samantha her feelings about being so dirty? Does Samantha feel comfortable about asking to be washed? Does Marion explain fully what a bed bath means and will Samantha be happy for her to carry this out?

Woman-centred care

Marion carries out a woman-centred approach to care and recognizes that Samantha is probably feeling weak and very tired after the birth of her baby at home. Marion has probably been with her for a long time too and recognizes the exhaustion Samantha is feeling. Questions that may arise include: What are Samantha's individual circumstances? What are her personal views of hygiene? Are there any religious beliefs that affect her views of hygiene? Are there underlying conditions that may affect her ability to get into a bath? Does Samantha wish to wash herself or give the responsibility to Marian?

Using best evidence

In this situation providing effective care will be based on clinical judgement as there is minimal research evidence as to the best forms of hygiene following a birth. However, some questions arise regarding mobility issues: How long will Samantha remain in bed? What underlying conditions may be affecting her skin integrity and recovery? What advice may be given to her to prevent the development of pressure ulcers or deep vein thrombosis?

Professional and legal issues

Midwives must practise within a professional and legal framework. Questions that may arise from this scenario are: Is Marion using her clinical judgement appropriately? Are there any health and safety issues in a midwife carrying out a bed bath at home? Are there any effects of her offering this service on her workload or on that of her colleague? Has Samantha consented to the procedure? Is there a documented plan of care? Has this been effectively evaluated?

Team working

In this situation there may be others who are supporting Marion at the home birth, and this could also be applied in a hospital setting. Are there any other team members who could carry out a bed bath instead? Is there a partner available who she would like to help or carry this out? If the midwife is concerned about Samantha's immobility or skin integrity who else should she refer to? Does the documentation support effective team working?

Clinical dexterity

The process of bathing in bed is covered above and the equipment required will be individual to each woman. In the home situation Marion will use the equipment that is available to her there. The skills required for bathing involve communication and psychological care as well as the physical requirements of the task. Questions that may arise are: If others are now carrying out bed baths how will students gain the skills to carry this out? What are the attitudes that are required by a midwife for this skill?

Models of care

Midwives will generally carry out bed baths and care of the immobile woman in a hospital setting. However, as in this scenario, it may need to be done in a home as well. The current changes in skill mix may lead to more maternity care assistants carrying out services such as these. However, midwives will still be involved in the supervision, teaching and giving assistance for bed baths. In this scenario questions arise such as: Who else on the team is available to support in this procedure? What are the benefits of 'total client care' rather than 'task led care'?

Safe environment

There is a minimal risk of a woman fainting in the bath; however, Marion's assessment of Samantha's wishes and her obvious tiredness may weigh against using a bath at home where there is no available equipment to raise her out in

case of collapse. Questions that may arise are: What are the facilities available in the home? Is there a suitable shower unit with a chair that could be utilized? What are the safety factors for the midwife carrying out a bed bath? Where is the source of hot water and is it safe to carry it to Samantha's bedside?

Promotes health

Midwives have an opportunity with each encounter to promote health and wellbeing for the woman and her family. In this situation Samantha has blood, liquor and meconium on her body from the skin-to-skin contact she has had with Jessica. Apart from the psychological unpleasantness of being 'messy' following the birth, there may also be concern because visitors may soon come to see the new family. Further, there is a minor risk of the spread of infection through the contamination. Questions that arise are: How may Marion use this opportunity to promote health and wellbeing on hygiene and mobility issues? What are the facilities for cleanliness in the home? What expectations do Samantha and her partner have of cleanliness? How can Marion demonstrate good hygiene practices in her care of Samantha and Jessica?

Further scenarios

The following scenarios enable you to consider how specific situations influence the care the midwife provides. Consider the following in relation to the jigsaw model.

Scenario 1

Ellen is transferred to the postnatal ward during the night. She has had a long and difficult labour which has ended with an emergency caesarean section of her first child. She is exhausted and uncomfortable.

Practice point

The midwife should weigh up the needs of the woman to rest following a long period in labour with the need to ensure that her hygiene and mobility needs are met. This is compounded by this being night time when there are often fewer members of staff available to carry out personal care.

Questions

- What is the impact of Ellen's birth experience on her mobility needs?
- What pain relief could be provided to enable Ellen to be encouraged to move regularly?
- What are the priorities that should be considered in ensuring Ellen's comfort?
- When would be the best time to meet Ellen's personal hygiene needs?
- What facilities are required near Ellen's bed space to ensure appropriate infection control?

Scenario 2

Maria is admitted to the antenatal ward with placenta praevia. She has had cerebral palsy since birth and is a wheelchair user.

Practice point

The midwife will need to consider both Maria's short-term and long-term requirements for hygiene and mobility.

- How will the midwife establish Maria's needs?
- What are Maria's hygiene and mobility needs?
- How may the ward team care for her appropriately?
- What equipment may be required to give effective care?
- Are there permanent family or carers who could provide support?

Conclusion

It is essential that, despite caring generally for fit and healthy women, midwives must recognize the importance of hygiene and mobility. Midwives should have an awareness of those women most at risk of damage to their skin and of the ways in which this is prevented. They should also have an awareness of the benefits and necessity of good hygiene practices.

Useful resources

Handwashing

http://www.npsa.nhs.uk/cleanyourhands

http://www.jr2.ox.ac.uk/bandolier/booth/booths/hand.html

http://www.rcn.org.uk/__data/assets/pdf_file/0003/78654/002741.pdf

Pressure area care

http://www.bbc.co.uk/health/conditions/pressuresores1.shtml

http://www.supplychain.nhs.uk/portal/page/portal/Products%20new/Pressure%20area%20care

http://www.rcn.org.uk/__data/assets/pdf_file/0003/109839/002166.pdf

Disabled parents

http://www.directgov.gov.uk/en/DisabledPeople/Disabledparents/index.htm

http://www.disabledparentsnetwork.org.uk/

http://www.dppi.org.uk/

References

Crowcroft N S, Catchpole M 2002 Mortality from methicillin resistant *Staphylococcus aureus* in England and Wales: analysis of death certificates. BMJ 325: 1390–1391

Department of Health 2004 Maternity Standard, National Service Framework for children, young people and maternity services. Department of Health, London

Department of Health 2006 The Health Act 2006 – Code of Practice for the prevention and control of health care associated infections. Department of Health, London

Healthcare Commission 2006 State of health care 2006. Commission for Healthcare Audit and Inspection, London

Morison B, Baker C 2001 How to raise awareness of pressure sore prevention. British Journal of Midwifery 9(3): 147–150

National Patient Safety Agency 2004 Clean your hands. Online. Available: http://www.npsa.nhs.uk/cleanyourhands 18 Apr 2007

NHS Modernisation Agency 2003a Essence of care: patient-focused benchmarks for clinical governance. Department of Health, London. Online. Available: http://www.cgsupport.nhs.uk/About_the_CGST/1@ Current_Work/Essence_of_Care_ Programme/The_Eleven_Benchmarks.asp 18 Feb 2008

NHS Modernisation Agency 2003b Benchmarks for personal and oral hygiene. Department of Health, London. Online. Available: http://www.cQsupport.nhs.uk/ downloads/Essence of Care/Personal & Oral Hygiene.doc 11 Nov 2006

NHS Modernisation Agency 2003c Benchmarks for pressure ulcers. Department of Health, London. Online. Available: http://www.cgsupport.nhs.uk/downloads/Essence of Care/Pressure Ulcers.doc 11 Nov 2006

Nursing and Midwifery Council (NMC) 2008 The Code. Standards of conduct, performance and ethics for nurses and midwives. NMC, London

Nursing and Midwifery Council (NMC) 2005 Infection control advice. NMC, London. Online. Available: http://www.nmc-uk.org/aFrameDisplay. aspx?DocumentlD=1577 11 Nov 2006

Nursing and Midwifery Council (NMC) 2004 Standards of proficiency for pre-registration midwifery education. NMC, London

Rotter M L 1998 Semmelweis' sesquicentennial: a little-noted anniversary of handwashing. Current Opinion in Infectious Diseases 11(4): 457–460

Skewes S 1996 Skin care rituals that do more harm than good. American Journal of Nursing 96(10): 32–35

Stewart M 2005 'I'm just going to wash you down': sanitizing the vaginal examination. Journal of Advanced Nursing 51(6): 587–594

The Information Centre 2006 NHS Maternity Statistics, England: 2004–05. The Information Centre, London. Online. Available: http://www.ic.nhs.uk/pubs/ maternityeng2005/maternitystats06/fileh. 13 Nov 2006

Vohra R K, McCollum C N 1994 Fortnightly Review: Pressure sores. BMJ 309: 853–857

Waterlow, J. (2005). Waterlow card. Online. Available: http://www.judy-waterlow.co.uk/ downloads/Waterlow%20Score%20Card. pdf. 23 Apr 07

Wolf Z R 1997 Nursing students' experience bathing patients for the first time. Nurse Educator 22(2): 41–46

Xavier G 1999 Asepsis. Nursing Standard 13(36): 49–53

Zaninotto P, Wardle H, Stamatakis E et al 2006 Forecasting obesity to 2010. Joint Health Surveys Unit. Department of Health, London

Chapter 4

Blood pressure measurement

Introduction

There are many ways in which midwives monitor the wellbeing of clients. The group of skills that involves measuring physical characteristics are often referred to as 'observations', one of which is blood pressure measurement. The measurement of blood pressure provides valuable information about a woman's health. It can be used to monitor her body's response to pregnancy, labour and birth. It is often recorded as a baseline measure in each of these circumstances to enable the carer to detect changes that may result from disease or obstetric intervention. Thus the midwife needs to understand what influences a woman's blood pressure, how to measure blood pressure accurately and the significance of the observation made.

Trigger scenario

Consider the following scenario in relation to the measurement of blood pressure. Try to identify what you need to know in order to interpret this situation.

Suzie's heart was pounding. The cuff felt tight and uncomfortable on her arm and then mercifully began to deflate. The midwife looked intently at the machine, listening. She then turned to the woman and said, 'That's fine'.

The following questions might have come to mind:

- Why is the midwife taking her blood pressure?
- How does the heart affect blood pressure, why was her heart pounding?
- What is a cuff, how is it applied and inflated, when is it deflated?
- Why was the cuff uncomfortable, what could be done to avoid discomfort?
- What is the machine called, what does it measure, are there different types, which is best?
- What is the midwife listening to, how does she listen, what does she use?
- How did the midwife know that the blood pressure was 'fine', what is normal?

You will find the answers to these questions within the chapter.

Definition

Blood pressure can be defined as: 'the force exerted by the blood on the vessel walls' (Johnson & Taylor 2006:55).

Background physiology

The circulatory system

Blood flow through the circulatory system is made possible due to the blood pressure gradient; blood pressure is highest near to the heart in the arteries and reduces as the blood flows away from the heart to the arterioles and the venous system.

The heart

Activity

Revise the anatomy and physiology of the heart. Ensure that you know what is meant by:

atrium, ventricle, sinoatrial node, atrioventricular node, bundle of His, Purkinje fibres, systole, diastole, stroke volume, heart rate.

The vascular and arterial systems

Systemic circulation

Blood rich in oxygen leaves the left ventricle of the heart via the aorta. The aorta divides into arteries and subdivides further into arterioles then capillaries. It is in the capillaries that exchange of gases, metabolic waste and nutrients takes place. The capillaries join to form venules, which further unite to form veins. Blood eventually returns to the right atrium of the heart from the lower body via the inferior vena cava and from the upper body via the superior vena cava.

Pulmonary circulation

Deoxgenated blood leaves the right ventricle of the heart via the pulmonary artery. This artery divides into two branches delivering the blood to the lungs, where the vessels divide into arterioles and capillaries as in the systemic circulation. Oxygenated blood is collected in venules and veins returning to the left side of the heart via four pulmonary veins.

Structure of blood vessels

All blood vessels comprise three layers, except capillaries, which are made of a single epithelial layer. The layers are:

Tunica intima – the inner layer made up of a single layer of endothelial cells.

Tunica media – the middle layer made up of elastic tissue and smooth muscle. In the aorta this layer is mostly elastic tissue with some muscle but as the arteries become smaller the proportion changes to become mostly muscle. In the venous system the vessel wall is thinner and more distensible, thus the veins are capable of carrying about 60% of the circulating blood volume (Stables & Rankin 2005).

Tunica adventicia – the outer layer made up of fibrous connective tissue.

Control of blood pressure

The blood pressure must be capable of responding to the demands of the body, and will vary accordingly. A range of factors influence arterial pressure including:

Cardiac output – (stroke volume × heart rate). Increased cardiac output leads to an increase in blood pressure, for example, during exercise. Cardiac output is also increased in response to sympathetic nerve stimulation following stress.

Arteriole peripheral resistance – The arteriole walls contain smooth muscle. When this smooth muscle contracts the lumen of the vessel decreases and the blood pressure increases. When smooth muscle relaxes the lumen of the vessel increases and the blood pressure is reduced. The renin-angiotensin system, which is stimulated in response to underperfusion of the glomerular apparatus in the kidney, leads to constriction of the arterioles and hence a rise in blood pressure.

Blood volume – A reduction in blood volume leads to a reduction in blood pressure, for example following haemorrhage. Although blood volume increases in pregnancy this does not lead to an increase in blood pressure because of reduced arteriole peripheral resistance.

Blood viscosity – Increased viscosity due to an increased number of red blood cells or plasma proteins leads to increased blood pressure. Severe anaemia could lead to reduced blood pressure.

The impact of pregnancy on blood pressure

During pregnancy there is an increase in cardiac output and circulating blood volume. However, due to the impact of progesterone relaxing the smooth muscle within the blood vessel walls, peripheral arteriole resistance is reduced and blood pressure remains within normal limits. There is virtually no change in systolic pressure during pregnancy but the diastolic pressure tends to reduce in the first two trimesters and return to pre-pregnancy values during the third trimester (Stables & Rankin 2005).

Most women have normal blood pressure throughout pregnancy, however, hypertensive disease in pregnancy is a significant cause of maternal death, resulting in 18 deaths in the 3-year period covered by the latest confidential enquiry (Lewis 2008). Although some women already have some degree of hypertensive disease, there is a pregnancy-specific disorder, called pre-eclampsia, that affects approximately 7% of all pregnancies (Sibai 1998). Pre-eclampsia may lead to serious complications in the mother including renal and hepatic failure, clotting disorders and haemorrhage and the baby may suffer the consequences of intrauterine growth restriction or premature birth (Enkin et al 2000).

The effects of pre-eclampsia can be minimized through prompt action. It is therefore vital that the woman's blood pressure is carefully assessed throughout the antenatal period so that appropriate care and treatment can be initiated if hypertension is discovered. Box 4.1 provides some working definitions developed by APEC for use in the care of women with hypertension in pregnancy.

Activity

Find out what social, psychologial and environmental factors impact on blood pressure and consider their relevance to pregnancy, labour and the postnatal period.

During labour, blood pressure rises due to the increased cardiac output asssociated with the physical exertion involved and exacerbated by pain and anxiety. Each contraction of the uterus adds 300–500 ml to the circulating volume (Stables & Rankin 2005). Postnatally the blood pressure should return to pre-labour values.

Box 4.1   Definitions of hypertension in pregnancy

Hypertension:	A diastolic blood pressure of 90 mmHg or above
Pre-existing hypertension:	Hypertension that existed pre-pregnancy or at booking (before 20 weeks)
New hypertension:	Hypertension at or after 20 weeks of pregnancy
Pre-eclampsia:	New hypertension and the presence of significant proteinurea (greater than or equal to 300 mg per 24 hours) at or after 20 weeks of pregnancy.

(PRECOG 2004:7)

National guidelines

NICE guidance (NICE 2008) recommends that blood pressure is measured at each antenatal visit, which for primigravida means a minimum of 10 recordings. The intervals for this observation are: ideally before 10 weeks, 16, 25, 28, 31, 34, 36, 38 and 40 weeks of pregnancy. Women who have already had a baby would have a minimum of seven antenatal checks, missing out a check at 25, 31 and 40 weeks of pregnancy.

The NICE Intrapartum Care Guidelines (NICE 2007) stipulate that the woman's blood pressure should be recorded when labour is first suspected and 4-hourly during the first stage of labour. Once the second stage of labour has been diagnosed the recommendation is that blood pressure is recorded hourly and then again after the baby is born.

The NICE Postnatal Care Guidelines (NICE 2006) recommend that the woman's blood pressure should be recorded within 6 hours of the birth, as a minimum. If the diastolic reading is greater than 90 mmHg it should be repeated in 4 hours. If it does not fall within this time the woman should be assessed for pre-eclampsia.

The charity Action on Pre-Eclampsia (APEC) have produced a *Pre-Eclampsia Community Guideline* (PRECOG) for use in the community which is endorsed by the Royal Colleges of Midwives, Obstetricians and General Practitioners and the National Childbirth Trust (see resources).

Activity

Raised blood pressure is a feature of pre-eclampsia. What are the other features of pre-eclampsia that the midwife might observe during an antenatal check?

Professional guidelines

To practise midwifery in the United Kingdom, midwives must work within the professional framework of the Nursing and Midwifery Council.

The activities of a midwife as described in the *Midwives rules and standards* (NMC 2004a, pp 36–37) include:

…monitor normal pregnancies…to recognize the warning signs of abnormality in the mother…monitor progress of the mother in the postnatal period.

All activities undertaken must be documented in accordance with the NMC *Guidelines for records and record keeping* (NMC 2005).

Activity

Access the *Standards of proficiency for pre-registration midwifery education* (NMC 2004b) and *The Code. Standards of conduct, performance and ethics* (NMC 2008). Consider which standards are relevant to the issue of observing pulse and respirations.

The measurement of blood pressure

The measurement of blood pressure, using the brachial artery in the arm, reflects arterial pressure. The pressure the blood exerts on the artery walls when the ventricles of the heart contract is called *systolic* pressure. It is measured in millimetres (mm) of mercury (Hg) and is normally in the range of 100–140 mmHg. The pressure the blood exerts on the artery walls when the ventricles relax is called *diastolic* pressure and this is normally in the range of 60–90 mmHg. Blood pressure is recorded systolic over diastolic and therefore a 'normal' blood pressure would be recorded as 120/75 mmHg.

Methods of measuring blood pressure

Blood pressure is measured using either the oscillatory or the auscultatory method.

Oscillatory method

The development of oscillatory or automatic devices is big business with a range of appliances available both for home and hospital use. Although there are automated devices that accurately measure blood pressure during pregnancy, a meta-analysis of validation studies of such devices showed that they under-read by clinically significant amounts in women with pre-eclampsia (Shennan & Waugh 2003). Whenever there is concern about a value given by an automated device the blood pressure should be checked again using the auscultatory method described below.

Auscultatory method

The traditional method for measuring blood pressure is by auscultation of the flow of blood through the brachial artery at the antecubital fossa. The instrument used to give a value to the sounds heard is called a sphygmomanometer and the instrument used to make the sounds audible is called a stethoscope.

Equipment

There are two methods of measuring blood pressure using the auscultatory method: the mercury and aneroid sphygmomanometers.

Mercury sphygmomanometer – This type of manometer has mercury contained in a glass column, with ascending numbers either side of the column. The column of mercury needs to be upright and the level observed at eye level. It is the most accurate method giving consistent readings and is heralded as the 'gold standard' for accurate blood pressure measurement (Valler-Jones & Wedgbury 2005). However, it is bulky, heavy and contains mercury which is hazardous to health. The Medicines and Healthcare products Regulatory Agency (MHRA) released a bulletin from the Medical Devices Agency (MDA 2000, p 4) advising the NHS to consider substituting mercury devices with alternative mercury-free products when the 'opportunity arises'. Many NHS Trusts have replaced their mercury syphgmomanometers with aneroid instruments.

Aneroid sphygmomanometer – This type of manometer has a circular gauge encased in glass, with a needle that points to numbers. These are lightweight, compact and portable but less accurate than the mercury devices. They should be re-calibrated on a regular basis.

Inflation cuff – Sphygmomanometers work using the principle of a bladder within a cuff being inflated around the upper arm to occlude the flow of blood through the brachial artery. The bladder is then gradually deflated by means of a valve in a hand held pump, until the blood flows through the artery again. This blood flow makes a noise that is heard (auscultated) through a stethoscope. These sounds are called Korotkoff sounds (Guyton 1997). The midwife listens to the Korotkoff sounds (see Table 4.1) and observes the dial of the aneroid device (or column of mercury) to measure the blood pressure.

The evidence relating to the measurement of blood pressure concludes that using an appropriate sized cuff is crucial for an accurate assessment of blood pressure. One study involving 1240 obese subjects (Maxwell 1982) found that using a standard

sized cuff on a large arm can give rise to false positive readings (raised blood pressure measurement when it is in fact normal). Conversely, using a large cuff on an average sized arm can create false negative readings (low blood pressure when it is in fact normal). A standard cuff should be used on women with an arm circumference of 33 cm or less.

The stethoscope – Most stethoscopes have earpieces connected by a long rubber tube to a bell-diaphragm end. It is this end piece that is placed over the artery so that the Korotkoff sounds can be auscultated. Although the bell end is more accurate, the diaphragm enables a wider area to be covered and is easier for the novice practitioner to secure in place.

Activity

Practise placing the earpiece in your ears and rotating the end piece in order to listen through the bell and then the diaphragm.

Korotkoff sounds

Korotkoff described five sounds audible through the stethoscope as the bladder in the cuff is deflated (Table 4.1).

Current consensus is that K5 is the measurement that should be recorded. Brown et al (1998) concluded from a randomized trial of 220 hypertensive pregnant women that K5 should be adopted as the diastolic blood pressure in pregnancy rather than K4, as the difference between the sounds is smaller in hypertensive pregnant women than those with a normal blood pressure. Consistency of approach to measurement is the most important clinical issue (Seifer, Samuals & Kniss 2001).

Table 4.1 Korotkoff sounds

Korotkoff phase	Sound heard through the stethoscope
1 Systolic pressure	First faint tapping sounds that gradually become louder
2	Sounds become fainter again but more swishing
Auscultatory gap	Sounds may disappear for a short time in some clients
3	Return of clear sounds again, may be even louder than K1
4	Sudden muffling of sounds that are softer in intensity
5 Diastolic pressure	Sounds have completely disappeared

The auscultatory gap

It is important that students are aware of this phenomenon because failure to take measures to identify the true systolic pressure could lead to K3 being recorded inadvertently. When measuring a client's blood pressure, the brachial pulse should be palpated before the stethoscope is applied to the arm. The cuff should be inflated about 30 mmHg above the pressure at which the pulse disappears. The cuff should then be deflated gradually and the pressure at which the pulse reappears is noted.

Now see where the auscultatory gap estimation fits into the whole procedure for auscultatory blood pressure measurement.

Undertaking blood pressure measurement

The protocol for measuring blood pressure has been described below. However, there is more to making a clinical observation than following a recipe; the woman's individual circumstances need to be taken into account. Any procedure, no matter how familiar to the practitioner, may

provoke anxiety or concern for the client.

Some women will accept the procedure as part of their care, but remain mildly stressed before each measurement. For other women, however, there may be unpleasant associations with the measurement of blood pressure. The midwife can easily ascertain how the woman feels about having her blood pressure measured simply by taking a moment to ask her. Women who have previously had children will have had their blood pressure measured previously. For those women who have never had their blood pressure taken before, a simple explanation of the procedure is required in order to alleviate any unnecessary concern.

1. The midwife discusses the procedure with the woman enabling her to understand its relevance to her care and give consent

The woman should be involved in decisions about her plan of care. For example, it should have been explained to her how often she will have her

Box 4.2   Procedure for blood pressure measurement

- **Consult the client's plan of care**
  Rationale To ensure effective monitoring of the client's condition. Clients should be sufficiently involved in their care that they are expecting to have their blood pressure checked

- **Gain verbal consent from the client**
  Rationale Consent for this procedure is often implied by an outstretched arm. However, it is courteous to ask before attempting to take a blood pressure measurement, and to talk to women who appear to be asleep

- **Locate sphygmomanometer, appropriate sized cuff and stethoscope**
  Rationale Gathering all equipment prior to the procedure avoids the need to leave the client during the consultation. The bladder in the cuff should go round 80% of the arm

- **Explain procedure if first time for client**
  Rationale The woman may have misconceptions requiring clarification

- **Client should be sitting or lying on side**
  Rationale To avoid vena-caval compression

- **The arm should be at the level of the heart and extended**
  Rationale If the arm is below the heart blood pressure may be overestimated. If the arm is above the heart the blood pressure may be underestimated

- **Tight sleeves should be removed**
  Rationale To ensure that blood is moving unimpeded through the vessels

- **Palpate brachial artery**
  Rationale To identify location of artery and point of maximum pulsation

- **Apply cuff over brachial artery, 2–3 cm above point of pulsation, rubber tubes uppermost**
  Rationale To ensure optimum auscultation of blood flow and easy access to artery

- **Re-palpate the brachial artery; rapidly pump cuff 20–30 mmHg above the pressure at which the pulse disappears. Deflate cuff gradually and note the pressure at which the pulse reappears (estimated systolic blood pressure)**
  Rationale To identify the approximate systolic blood pressure and avoid underestimation by avoiding the auscultatory gap

- **Apply stethoscope using the diaphragm side**
  Rationale To listen to the blood flow in the artery over maximum area

- **Close valve on bulb with forefinger and thumb in clockwise rotation and pump up cuff observing pressure gauge, until 20–30 mmHg above estimated systolic pressure**
  Rationale To inflate cuff to occlude blood flow, avoiding overinflation and unnecessary discomfort

- **Slowly release valve (anticlockwise rotation) at rate of 2 mmHg per second and note when the sounds return**
  Rationale To identify systolic blood pressure

continued

Box 2.2 continued

- **Continue listening until all sound disappears**
  Rationale To identify diastolic blood pressure

- **Release the valve completely and remove the cuff**
  Rationale To ensure client comfort

- **Assist the client to rearrange her clothes, if appropriate**
  Rationale To maintain client dignity and comfort

- **Inform the client of the value measured and the significance**
  Rationale To involve the client in her care

- **Record the result in the woman's notes**
  Rationale To ensure continuity, completeness and compliance with professional standards.

---

blood pressure checked and in what circumstances that plan might change. She should understand how her individual circumstances have informed the plan of care. The midwife can also use the opportunity to convey to the woman the importance of reporting other symptoms of pre-eclampsia. If the woman asks any questions about the procedure these should be answered with confidence or referred to someone else who can answer.

It is important that midwives seek and gain consent for any procedure, no matter how routine. S/he should understand what the procedure involves and the significance of the results.

2. The observation is made at the appropriate time according to the woman's plan of care

Blood pressure is usually measured at the booking visit and at every subsequent antenatal examination in accordance with the national antenatal care guidelines (NICE 2008). However, some women will require additional measurements because of their previous history or due to a change in condition, and this plan should be documented in the notes.

Activity

Think about how this changes for women in the following circumstances: with an epidural in situ, following caesarean birth, woman on medication for hypertension in the postnatal period.

The timing of the measurement in relation to other events is also important. For example, it is recommended that a pregnant woman should have her blood pressure taken after a period of rest (Precog 2004). When measuring blood pressure during labour, it should only be taken in-between contractions due to the increased cardiac output during contractions.

Activity

Try to find out how timing affects the blood pressure measurement in relation to: recent activity, consumption of food, smoking, drinking caffeine, morning/evening.

3. The observation is made using the correct technique

Practitioners should familiarize themselves with the use of electronic blood pressure equipment when they have achieved competence with the more traditional equipment. As there is a range of electronic products in use, the midwife must make herself familiar with new equipment and attend training provided by employers regarding its use.

4. The woman is supported during the observation and her reaction observed

Blood pressure measurement is a short and non-invasive procedure and the woman should not require additional support. You will not be able to talk while you are listening and should therefore ensure that the woman knows that you are not ignoring her, but concentrating hard on what you can hear. Taking a woman's blood pressure should not induce any untoward response in the woman, although she may be anxious about the result. You will not be able to look at her face during the procedure but can ascertain that her arm is comfortable immediately following the measurement.

Activity

What is meant by the term 'white coat hypertension'? Think about what the midwife can do to help avoid it.

5. The woman is made comfortable after the measurement

Where clothing had been removed to gain access to the arm, care should be taken to ensure that the woman's dignity is maintained and she is not unduly exposed. Where the woman is having automated blood pressure measurements taken at intervals, her comfort should be regularly reassessed.

6. The woman is informed of the result

It should be the practitioner's common practice to convey results to clients. The value should be given, so that the client becomes familiar with what is normal for her, followed by an interpretation. Questions are most likely to arise following the measurement of blood pressure in relation to whether it is normal or not. Any uncertainty relating to questions asked must be referred to a senior colleague for clarification.

7. If the result is outside normal parameters it is reported to an appropriate member of the team

Students must be able to recognize the importance of blood pressure monitoring during pregnancy, labour and the puerperium and be prepared to seek help from a registered practitioner if they are in any doubt about a measurement or its significance. Having recorded the blood pressure the student must inform a registered practitioner of her findings.

Activity

List two of the complications of raised blood pressure in pregnancy.

8. An accurate and legible record is made of the observation

The blood pressure measurement is recorded as a fraction with the systolic reading above the diastolic. It should be dated and timed, written in black ink and counter-signed by a registered practitioner. Where any action was taken as a result of the measurement, this should also be documented and a plan of care developed.

Reflection on trigger scenario

Look back at the trigger scenario.

Suzie's heart was pounding. The cuff felt tight and uncomfortable on her arm and then mercifully began to deflate. The midwife looked intently at the machine, listening. She then turned to the woman and said, 'That's fine'.

It could have described Suzie's experience of having her blood pressure taken at any point during her pregnancy, labour or postnatal care. Now that you are familiar with the physiology of blood pressure and the way that it is monitored you should have more insight into the description of the midwife's behaviour in that short extract. The jigsaw model will now be used to explore the trigger scenario in more depth.

Effective communication

Effective verbal and non-verbal communication is fundamental to the provision of sensitive midwifery care. We need to be aware of the way we are presenting ourselves when caring for women. Questions that arise from the scenario might include: has the midwife already explained what she is doing and why? Is she aware that the woman may feel ignored during the procedure? How can this be avoided? Did she go on to explain the result to the woman? If so, how did she do this? Did she show Suzie the record she made in her notes and explain it?

Woman-centred care

Providing sensitive and individualized care necessitates engaging with the woman, involving her in her care and providing her with feedback. Questions that arise from the scenario might include: Why was Suzie's heart pounding? What are her individual circumstances? How has the midwife taken these into account? How has the midwife involved Suzie in her care? How has her assessment been tailored to her individual needs? Has Suzie ever had raised blood pressure? Does she have a family history of hypertension?

Using best evidence

To provide effective care to women the midwife must use her knowledge regarding the most appropriate means and method for measuring blood pressure in the circumstances. Questions that arise from the scenario might include: What kind of machine is the midwife using? Is it the most appropriate equipment in the circumstances? When was it last calibrated? Did she palpate the pulse at the antecubital fossa? Did she use the appropriate cuff size? Where was the arm positioned? Did she pump the cuff 30 mmHg above the pressure at which the pulse disappears to avoid the auscultatory gap?

Professional and legal issues

Midwives must practise within a professional and legal framework to maintain high standards of care and protect women from potential harm. To evaluate the scenario further you might consider the following issues: Where does it state that it is the midwife's role to monitor a woman's condition? Did the midwife ask Suzie's consent before she took her blood pressure? Did she explain why she was taking her blood pressure? What should the midwife do if the result was abnormal?

Team working

It only takes one person to take a blood pressure but a whole host of professionals become involved when pre-eclampsia is suspected. Questions that arise from the scenario might include: Who else can monitor blood pressure in the maternity setting? If an abnormal blood pressure had been detected, who else should have been involved? What is the process for referring a pregnant woman with high blood pressure for further investigation? How would this differ in the postnatal period? How can midwives facilitate effective team working?

Clinical dexterity

Using the auscultatory method for measuring blood pressure requires a certain degree of dexterity. Not only does the student need to manipulate the valve on the cuff's bladder but they also need to listen to the sound and watch the dial at the same time. Achieving dexterity takes practice. Questions that arise from the scenario might include: Is the midwife having difficulty hearing the Korotkoff sounds? How will I be able to do this quickly in-between the contractions of a labouring woman?

Models of care

Midwives take blood pressure in a range of settings. How care is organized is likely to influence the way that blood pressure is measured. Questions that arise from the scenario might include: Where is Suzie when her blood pressure is being monitored? Is she close to home or has she travelled large distances, coping with public transport or congested car parks in order to have her blood pressure measured? How will the model of care she is experiencing influence the subsequent care she receives? Who is at hand to support the midwife who is providing care?

Safe environment

Midwives work in a variety of locations and need to assess the risks each environment poses. Ensuring that the woman will not come to any harm during the procedure is paramount. Blood pressure measurement is a non-invasive procedure and is not a risk to a woman's wellbeing. However, if the woman needs to undress in any way in order to provide an unrestricted arm for the procedure, she is at risk of losing dignity. If she is asked to lie flat on her back for the procedure she may be at risk of vena-caval compression and subsequently low blood pressure. Questions that arise from the scenario might include: Is the equipment appropriately maintained? Is it positioned correctly for optimum comfort of the woman and the midwife? Has the woman's dignity been maintained throughout the procedure? Did the midwife wash her hands in between clients?

Promotes health

Routine antenatal care provides many opportunities to promote the health and wellbeing of both the woman and her family. Questions that arise from the scenario might include: Did the midwife explain the significance of raised blood pressure during pregnancy? If the woman was pregnant, did the midwife describe the signs and symptoms of pre-eclampsia so that the woman knows when to self-refer? Does the woman know how to get in touch with her midwife? Similarly, if the woman was postnatal, did the woman understand when to contact a health professional if symptoms of hypertension developed?

Further scenarios

The following scenarios enable you to consider how specific situations influence the care the midwife provides. Use the jigsaw model to explore the issues raised in each scenario.

Scenario 1

Lucy is 15 years old and 12 weeks pregnant. She has come to the antenatal clinic for the first time accompanied by her mother. Every time you ask Lucy a question her mother answers it for her. You ask her if it would be ok to take her blood pressure and her mother says, 'Yes, you'd better check it. I had toxaemia when I was having her'.

Practice point

Not all pregnant teenagers have the support of their parents throughout their pregnancy. However, midwives need to employ strategies to facilitate the development of woman-centred care whilst ensuring that the mother is not alienated or sidelined. The mother is a valuable source of information regarding the teenager's family and medical history and will continue to have a role in her life, long after the midwife has fulfilled hers.

Further questions specific to Scenario 1 include:

- Did the midwife explain the reason for taking blood pressure at every antenatal visit?
- Did the midwife explain the procedure as this was Lucy's first antenatal visit?

- How would you explain the procedure to a 15-year-old? Does age make a difference to the explanation given?
- Did she use her knowledge of the importance of family history in assessing Lucy's risk of pre-eclampsia?
- What strategies could the midwife use to ensure that Lucy remained the focus of her care, whilst involving her mother appropriately?

Scenario 2

Tessa is in labour. She is in the birthing pool and coping well with her contractions. She wants to change position and stands up. She suddenly feels faint.

Practice point

Water provides many benefits to the woman including the analgesic and relaxing effects of the warm water, but there are also some unexpected potential hazards that can be avoided through simple preventative measures. Women who labour in water should not be left alone at any time.

Further questions specific to Scenario 2 include:

- Why does Tessa feel faint when she stands up? How has the use of the birthing pool contributed to this?
- How can the midwife help Tessa to feel less faint?
- How often should Tessa's blood pressure be recorded?
- Where should Tessa's blood pressure be recorded?
- If Tessa decided that she wanted an epidural for pain relief how would this change her care in relation to blood pressure monitoring?

Conclusion

There are many factors that impact on blood pressure and the midwife must be aware of the relevance of these factors on pregnancy, labour and the postnatal period. There are also many considerations that the midwife must take into account in order to obtain accurate blood pressure readings. Although blood pressure measurement becomes a routine aspect of the midwife's clinical practice, she must be alert to the fact that each measurement she makes is a valuable piece of information, not only for her and the healthcare team but most importantly, for the woman.

Useful resources

Action on pre eclampsia
http://www.apec.org.uk/
Antenatal care: Routine care of the healthy pregnant woman. NICE guidance

http://www.nice.org.uk/guidance/CG62
British Hypertension Society
http://www.bhsoc.org/default.stm
http://www.abdn.ac.uk

References

Brown M A, Buddle M L, Farrell T et al 1998 Randomised trial of management of hypertensive pregnancies by Korotkoff phase IV or phase V. The Lancet 352: 777–781

Department of Health 1998 Report on the confidential enquiries into maternal deaths in the United Kingdom 1994–1996

Enkin M, Keirse M J N C, Neilson. J et al 2000 A guide to effective care in pregnancy and childbirth, 3rd edn. Oxford University Press, Oxford

Guyton A C, Hall J E 1997 Human physiology and mechanisms of disease, 6th edn. WB Saunders Company, Philadelphia

Johnson R, Taylor W 2006 Skills for midwifery practice, 2nd edn. Harcourt Health Science, Elsevier, Edinburgh

Lewis G. (Ed.) 2007 Saving Mothers' Lives. 2003–2005. Report of the 7th confidential enquiry into maternal death. CEMACH, London

Maxwell M, Waks A et al 1982 Error in blood pressure measurement due to incorrect cuff size in obese patients. Lancet 2: 33–36

Medical Device Agency (MDA) 2000 Devices Bulletin. Blood pressure measurement devices. Mercury and non-mercury. July

National Institute for Health and Clinical Excellence (NICE) 2006 Routine postnatal care of women and their babies. NICE clinical guideline 37. NICE, London

National Institute for Health and Clinical Excellence (NICE) 2007 Intrapartum care: care of healthy women and their babies during childbirth. NICE clinical guideline 55. RCOG Press, London

National Institute for Health and Clinical Excellence (NICE) 2008 Antenatal care: routine care for the healthy pregnant woman. Clinical guideline 62. RCOG Press, London

Nursing and Midwifery Council (NMC) 2004a Midwives rules and standards. NMC, London

Nursing and Midwifery Council (NMC) 2004b Standards of proficiency for pre-registration midwifery education. NMC, London

Nursing and Midwifery Council (NMC) 2005 Guidelines for records and record keeping. NMC, London

Nursing and Midwifery Council (NMC) 2008 The Code. Standards of conduct, performance and ethics for nurses and midwives. NMC, London.

Precog 2004 Pre-eclampsia community guideline. Action on pre-eclampsia

Seifer D B, Samuals P, Kniss D A 2001 The physiologic basis of gynaecology and obstetrics. Lippencott, Williams & Wilkins, Philadelphia

Shennan A, Waugh J 2003 The measurement of blood pressure and proteinurea. In: Critchley H, MacLean A, Poston L et al (eds) Pre-eclampsia. RCOG Press, London, pp 305–324

Sibai B M 1998 Prevention of pre-eclampsia: a big disappointment. American Journal of Obstetrics and Gynaecology 179: 1275–1278

Stables D, Rankin J (eds) 2005 Physiology in childbearing with anatomy and related biosciences, 2nd edn. Elsevier, Edinburgh

De Sweit M 2000 K5 rather than K4 for diastolic blood pressure measurement in pregnancy. Hypertension in Pregnancy 19(2): V–VII

Valler-Jones T, Wedgbury K 2005 Measuring blood pressure using the mercury sphygmomanometer. British Journal of Nursing 14(3): 145–150

Chapter 5

Temperature measurement

Introduction

Temperature measurement is one of the clinical observations, along with blood pressure, pulse and respiration rate, that is part of the activity known as 'doing the obs'. Together these observations provide valuable information about how well the body is adjusting to the clinical situation. The body as an organism needs to be able to maintain the appropriate temperature in whatever conditions it is situated. The measurement of the internal temperature is an important guide to the body's reaction to external conditions but also an indicator of the presence of internal problems, such as infection. The midwife needs to know how to measure temperature in the woman and the neonate, and to understand the significance of the observation.

Trigger scenario

Consider the following scenario in relation to the measurement of temperature and what you need to know to help you interpret the situation.

Julia had a caesarean section 2 days ago and was breastfeeding her baby. She was taking iron tablets for anaemia and analgesia for her wound, which was quite painful. Jessica, the student midwife, recorded Julia's temperature. It was 37.8°C. 'Is it normal?' Julia asked.

You may have thought of the following questions:

- What is the normal body temperature in adults and in neonates?
- How is temperature measured?
- How is temperature recorded?
- What does it mean if temperature falls outside the normal range?
- What factors may cause an abnormal reading?
- How might a caesarean section affect temperature?
- Does breastfeeding cause maternal temperature fluctuations?
- Should the student inform the woman if her temperature is abnormal?
- What else should the student do if she discovers an abnormal temperature?

Background physiology

Normal body temperature in adults

The normal core temperature in adults is 37°C. The core temperature is that of the brain and abdominal and chest organs (Johnson & Taylor 2006) and should remain constant despite changes in the external environment. Peripheral temperature fluctuates depending on the temperature of the external environment and there may be approximately 1°C difference between core and peripheral temperature (Blows 2001). The body seeks to maintain a core temperature of 37°C as this is optimum for the activity of the enzymes that regulate biochemical changes and physiological functions (Coad 2006).

Maintaining this optimum temperature is therefore a balance between heat production and heat dissipation. Heat is produced during cellular metabolism, particularly in the liver and muscle cells (Blows 2001) and is dissipated via the blood to the peripheries of the body. Temperature receptors in the skin detect changes in temperature and send nerve impulses to the cerebral cortex and hypothalamus in the brain. The hypothalamus also detects the temperature of the blood directly, as do sensors in some internal organs, the spinal cord and major blood vessels (Guyton & Hall 2007). The hypothalamus activates changes necessary to maintain the core temperature at 37°C.

When core temperature exceeds 38°C, this is termed pyrexia (Mallik et al. 1998). If the temperature rises above 37°C the sympathetic nervous system is activated and sweating or diaphoresis is induced, enabling the body to cool by a process of evaporation. Dilation of the peripheral skin vessels results in

blood being brought closer to the skin surface and heat is lost through radiation. Voluntary acts, like shedding clothes or drinking, are also activated.

Heat loss can be summarized as follows:

- *Radiation* – Heat transfer from hot object to cooler environment
- *Evaporation* – Escape of water and heat from the surface of a body
- *Convection* – Displacement of cooler air by rising hot air
- *Conduction* – Heat transfer from hot to cold touching objects.

Physiology in relation to pregnancy

Pregnant women often have warm hands and feet, due to a seven-fold increase in blood flow to the extremities (Coad 2006). The basal metabolic rate is raised, resulting in increased heat generation of up to 35% (Johnson & Taylor 2006) and an increase in maternal temperature of 0.5°C. Following childbirth temperature can be elevated to 38°C for 24 hours and this may be attributed to dehydration (McKinney et al 2000). Maternal temperature may also rise on the second or third days postnatally, when milk production begins and persists for a few days (Johnson & Taylor 2006).

Activity

Consider the above information and apply this to your practice situation.

Neonatal temperature regulation

A temperature of up to 37.2°C is acceptable for a baby in a neonatal unit or postnatal ward. A temperature below 36.5°C is considered hypothermic (Baston & Durward 2001). Coad (2006) describes how heat transfer is affected by two gradients: the internal gradient involves heat transfer from the core to the surface of the baby and the external gradient involves heat transfer from the body surface to the environment. Heat is lost rapidly at birth as the external environment is cooler than the uterus. The baby is also wet with amniotic fluid, evaporation of which leads to rapid cooling. Neonates have a high surface area to body weight ratio. The surface area from which they can lose heat is much larger than the body mass that can generate heat. They have less subcutaneous fat than adults, which means that their blood vessels are nearer the skin surface facilitating rapid transfer of heat from the core to the skin surface. The head is particularly prone to heat loss, comprising 25% of the neonate's surface area (Stables 2005).

oxygen and glucose. The neonate's natural attitude of flexion also helps prevent heat loss (Burroughs & Leifer 2001). Allowing the neonate to become cool is potentially lethal. A cold baby will utilize stores of glucose and increase its oxygen consumption in an attempt to increase its basal metabolic rate (BMR) through the metabolism of BAT. Eventually this process may result in low blood sugar (hypoglycaemia) and lack of oxygen to the tissues (hypoxia) leading to a lowering of blood pH (acidosis). The fatty acids released by the metabolism of brown fat can also interfere with the transportation of bilirubin to the liver resulting in hyperbilirubinaemia (McKinney et al 2000). The neonate is less well equipped to lose heat purposefully, peripheral vasodilatation being the main source of heat loss (Coad 2006). Although the neonate has sweat glands they are immature and limited in their capability to increase heat loss by evaporation.

Activity

Identify three reasons why a baby born before 37 completed weeks' gestation may be more vulnerable to heat loss. How can heat loss in the newborn infant be prevented?

Activity

Find out where brown adipose tissue is concentrated in the neonate. Explain the meaning of a neutral thermal environment.

The neonate can generate heat in response to a drop in environmental temperature. Brown adipose tissue (BAT), a highly vascular tissue packed with mitochondria, is stimulated to produce heat following the release of adrenaline and noradrenaline from the sympathetic nervous system. This form of thermogenesis is known as 'non-shivering thermogenesis' (NST) dependent on sufficient supplies of

National guidance

The National Service Framework for Children, Young People and Maternity Services (Department of Health 2004) stipulates the provision of individualized, woman-centred care which entails using appropriate observations for the appropriate situation. Further, there is the requirement for midwives to be able to recognize when a woman needs referral to other practitioners within the multi-professional team.

There is no specific guidance relating to pulse and respiration in the NICE guidelines for antenatal care (NICE 2008). In the NICE intrapartum guideline (NICE 2007) a woman's temperature should be taken as an observation when labour is suspected and then should be observed 4-hourly throughout labour and again after the birth. The baby's temperature should be recorded soon after the first hour of birth, after the baby has enjoyed skin to skin contact with his mother.

The postnatal care guideline (NICE 2006:12) states that:

In the absence of any signs and symptoms of infection, routine assessment of temperature is unnecessary.

- Temperature should be taken and documented if infection is suspected. If the temperature is above 38°C, repeat measurement in 4–6 hours.
- If the temperature remains above 38°C on the second reading or there are other observable symptoms and measurable signs of sepsis, evaluate further (emergency action).

There are also guidelines for the care of babies:

- They should have a temperature of 37°C in a normal room environment.
- The temperature of a baby does not need to be taken, unless there are specific risk factors, for example maternal pyrexia during labour.
- When a baby is suspected of being unwell, the temperature should be measured using electronic devices that have been properly calibrated and are used appropriately.
- A temperature of 38°C or more is abnormal and the cause should be

evaluated (emergency action). A full assessment, including physical examination, should be undertaken.

Professional guidelines

Activity

Access the Standards of proficiency for pre-registration midwifery education (NMC 2004a) and The Code. Standards of conduct, performance and ethics (NMC 2008). Consider which standards are relevant to the issue of taking temperature.

The Midwives rules (NMC 2004b:16) also cover the responsibility of midwives (Rule 6) to recognize deviation from normal in the woman or baby and to refer such cases to an appropriate health professional.

Site for temperature measurement

Choosing the most appropriate site for measurement of temperature must take into account the age, compliance and condition of the client and the instrument to be used.

Oral site

This has been the most common site of choice for clinical practice. However, it is not appropriate for clients who feel nauseous, are at risk of fainting or fitting, in pain or uncooperative. It is therefore unsuitable during labour and for babies and young children. The thermometer should be placed in the sublingual pocket (under the tongue at either side). Readings may be affected by recent hot or cold drinks and 15 minutes should be allowed to elapse if this site is chosen.

Activity

Find out what other factors impact on body temperature, including time of day, exercise, bathing, menstrual cycle and smoking.

Tympanic

With the development of electronic thermometers the use of the ear as a site has become more common. It is a generally acceptable site for all people, however there are mixed results reported from respective research on the accuracy of this method for both adults and children (Purssell 2007).

Axilla

This is the most appropriate site for taking the neonate's temperature. The thermometer should be positioned under the axilla, perpendicular to the chest wall and the arm held in place for the required length of time, depending on the manufacturer's guidelines for the type of thermometer in use. Any procedure involving the baby should avoid undue removal of clothing. The axilla is also the site of choice in clients whose condition renders them unable to tolerate an oral thermometer (see above) or who may inadvertently bite it.

Rectal site

This site for temperature estimation is not recommended for routine practice

due to the potential risk of trauma to the rectal mucosa in babies and embarrassment in adults.

Thermometers

There are a range of tools to enable the practitioner to measure temperature. Table 5.1 summarizes the site and method for each tool. The traditional glass and mercury thermometer is no longer in professional use. However, they may still be in use in the home, and practitioners should remind parents of the risks and hazards associated with glass breakage and mercury spillage.

Activity

Find out the type of thermometers in use locally and find out what research has been carried out into their use.

---

1. The midwife discusses the procedure with the woman enabling her to understand its relevance to her care and give consent

Any procedure, no matter how familiar to the practitioner, may cause anxiety in clients. Most women will have had their temperature taken before they reach childbearing age, but they may only be familiar with the mercury thermometer. Devices and their method of use should be explained. For example, to approach a woman saying, 'I'm just going to take your temperature' and then inserting an instrument into her ear, could be alarming for someone who has never encountered a tympanic thermometer. The practitioner can ascertain if the

Table 5.1 Choice of thermometer

Device	Site	Method	Considerations
Electronic	Oral, axilla	Cover probe with a disposable cover. Switch on and site. Alarm sounds after 1–2mins; reading taken	Clean and maintain according to manufacturer's instructions
Tympanic	Tympanic membrane	Apply disposable sheath. Switch on and insert in ear, sealing the auditory canal, read when alarm sounds	User must read instructions pertaining to specific instrument. Maintenance essential to ensure accuracy
Disposable	Oral, axilla	Remove from packet and peel back top of wrapper to expose handle. Remove from wrapper and site. Leave for 3 min then remove. Wait 10 s before reading. The last dot indicates the temperature. Dispose	Needs careful storage in optimum temperature. Sterile

Box 5.1 Procedure for temperature measurement

- **Consult the client's plan of care**
  Rationale To ensure effective monitoring of the client's condition. Clients should be sufficiently involved in their care that they are expecting to have their temperature taken

- **Gain verbal consent from the client**
  Rationale Consent for this procedure is often implied by an open mouth, lifted arm or hair tucked behind the ear. However, it is courteous to ask before attempting to take a client's temperature and to talk to women who appear to be asleep. Consent should also be gained

from parents before taking a baby's temperature

- **Ensure no recent activity that might impact on result**
  Rationale To achieve an accurate temperature reading

- **Locate the appropriate thermometer and ensure in working order**
  Rationale It is essential that the appropriate thermometer is chosen, depending on the client. Where the device is electronic it is important

continued

Box 5.1 continued

to check that it is operational before commencing the procedure to avoid leaving the prepared client during the activity

- **Explain the procedure if first time for client**
  Rationale Client may have misconceptions requiring clarification. There are many different types of thermometers used in clinical practice and the client may not be familiar with the instrument to be used

- **Client should be sitting or lying (on side if pregnant)**
  Rationale To avoid client falling. To avoid vena-caval compression, if pregnant

- **Close door or curtains if client is required to remove any clothing during access**
  Rationale To maintain client's privacy and dignity. To ensure draught free environment for neonate, thus avoiding further cooling

- **Apply thermometer in accordance with manufacturer's instructions**

  Rationale To achieve accurate temperature recording

- **Read the thermometer**
  Rationale To identify the client's temperature

- **Assist the client to rearrange her clothes, if appropriate**
  Rationale To maintain client comfort and dignity

- **The neonate must be left sufficiently wrapped**
  Rationale To ensure the neonate does not become cool as a result of the procedure

- **Inform the client of the value measured and the significance**
  Rationale To involve the client in her care and provide reassurance

- **Record the result in the woman's/baby's notes**
  Rationale To ensure continuity, completeness and compliance with professional standards.

woman is familiar with the procedure through simple questioning, avoiding inappropriately lengthy explanations. Increasingly, alternative devices will be used in women's homes as they are available for purchase in the high street.

Questions are likely to concern whether the temperature is normal. Midwives should therefore be familiar with normal temperature values for women and babies. The implications of abnormal values need careful explanation.

Activity

Draw a flowchart showing what a midwife should do if she detects a raised temperature in a woman who has had a normal vaginal birth the previous day.

Normal values should always be conveyed to the woman so that she becomes familiar with what is normal for her and feels that she is involved in her care.

2. The observation is made at the appropriate time according to the woman's plan of care

The midwife will use her professional judgement to identify when it is appropriate to take a client's temperature according to the individual client's condition. However, there are key points during the childbirth continuum when temperature should be assessed (Box 5.2).

The plan of care should be consulted regarding the timing and frequency of the measurement of temperature. For example, a baby may have become cool after birth and various measures may have been employed to bring the temperature back to normal prior to transfer. Instructions may have been written in the care plan as to the

---

Box 5.2 When to assess a client's temperature

Antenatal period

Any antenatal admission to hospital or physical cause for concern, including abdominal pain, labour, rupture of membranes, antepartum haemorrhage. This enables a baseline to be established and detection of possible infection requiring further investigation, for example in the urinary tract.

Intrapartum period

4-hourly during labour, unless evidence of pyrexia, in which case a doctor should be informed and temperature monitored hourly. Pyrexia may be a sign of dehydration or developing infection.

Postnatal period

Temperature is taken following birth and again before the attending midwife leaves the home (if a home birth) or transfers the woman's care to the postnatal ward.

NICE guidelines (2006) state that the woman's temperature should be taken if there are signs of infection. If above 38°C it should be measured again in 4–6 hours. If this is above 38°C or there is concern about her condition she should be referred immediately.

Following surgery a woman is more at risk of infection and her temperature will be monitored more frequently until the wound has healed. Assessment will also be made if there is any deterioration in her condition or where infection is suspected, for example painful wound, dysuria, abdominal tenderness, painful calf, mastitis.

Neonatal period

The baby's temperature is checked at the first physical examination by the midwife, soon after birth and again approximately an hour later to ensure the correct temperature is maintained. Temperature will be reassessed on transfer to the ward or home. NICE (2006) state that an electronic device should be used if there is suspicion of the baby being unwell and referral made if temperature is 38°C or above, repeated again 4–6 hours later.

frequency that the baby's temperature should be checked to ensure the temperature is maintained. Not doing so may put the baby at risk and could constitute negligence if harm came to the baby.

Activity

Identify your Trust's current policy regarding temperature monitoring for women after spontaneous rupture of membranes, normal vaginal birth and caesarean section.

3. The observation is made using the correct technique

The midwife should be familiar with all types of thermometers available in her area of work and should ensure the appropriate tool is used for the individual client. It is beneficial to use the same type for each measurement on each individual client in case of discrepancy in the calibration of a piece of equipment. Box 5.1 shows how to carry out temperature measurement.

4. The woman is supported during the observation and her reaction observed

Measuring a client's temperature is a relatively short procedure which should not cause discomfort or pain. If using an oral thermometer the practitioner should not ask the woman to talk, as it is not only difficult for the client but could also make the result inaccurate. When a baby's temperature is being taken the practitioner should endeavour to keep the baby warm and talk to the baby, acting as a role model to the new parents.

Taking a temperature should not induce any untoward response from either the woman or the baby, though if it is being taken due to concern about her wellbeing, or that of her baby, she may be feeling anxious and any anxieties should be explored. It may be that during the procedure other issues that need reporting may be detected or revealed. For example, while taking the baby's temperature the woman may raise concerns about breastfeeding or the baby's sleeping pattern. Adopting an unhurried and individualized approach to care will enable women to reveal and discuss their concerns.

5. The woman is made comfortable after the measurement

If clothing is removed to access the axilla, care should be taken to ensure that dignity is maintained and the woman helped to redress if appropriate. The baby should also be dressed and returned to the mother for comfort if required.

6. The woman is informed of the result

If the result is in the normal range this should be indicated to the woman. If the temperature is outside the normal range the significance of this should be explained to her carefully, especially in relation to her baby, as it may cause her anxiety.

7. If the result is outside normal parameters it is reported to an appropriate member of the team

As indicated above midwives should understand the significance of temperature ranges in both women and babies. If the values fall outside what is regarded as normal she should inform a registered practitioner of her findings.

8. An accurate and legible record is made of the observation

It is important that a client's condition can be monitored over time. Readings must be recorded on the appropriate documentation, usually in black ink, and where any action was taken as a result of the measurement, this should also be documented and a plan of care developed.

Activity

Find out in your Trust where temperatures are recorded for both mothers and babies.

Reflection on trigger scenario

Reconsider the trigger scenario at the beginning of the chapter:

Julia had a caesarean section two days ago and was breastfeeding her baby. She was taking iron tablets for anaemia and analgesia for her wound, which was quite painful. Jessica, the student midwife, recorded Julia's temperature. It was 37.8°C. 'Is it normal?' Julia asked.

The story concerns a woman following birth, and it is more likely that the issues of temperature recording will be in the postnatal period. However, any issues raised above should be applied to any situation where a woman shows signs of infection during pregnancy and beyond. This chapter has

explored some of the physiological and psychological issues around caring for women in this situation and you will have more insight into the issues in the scenario. The jigsaw model will be used to consider the issues in more depth.

Effective communication

In all situations in maternity care effective communication is important for the psychological wellbeing of the woman. In this situation where Julia has had a caesarean section recently she may be feeling tired and anxious as well as in pain following this major operation. The midwife should therefore be sensitive about how she communicates information to ensure Julia understands what is being said. Further, how Jessica records the information is important. Some questions that could arise are: Has Jessica been caring for Julia previous to this encounter or is it the first time they have met? What information should Jessica give prior to commencing the procedure? How did Julia ask the question? Is she showing signs of anxiety or excessive pain? How will Jessica answer the question? How will Jessica record the information obtained?

Woman-centred care

A woman-centred approach to this procedure would have been to look at the whole pattern of care required by Julia during that shift and assess when would be the best time to take her temperature and with what kind of thermometer. Further whole person assessment should be made in respect of the effect of operative birth and pain on temperature, and also the external temperature of the environment. Questions that may arise include: Is taking a temperature appropriate when she is breastfeeding? Has Jessica recently had a hot drink? Should something be done about her pain before taking a temperature? What is the most appropriate type of thermometer to use and is she familiar with its use? What other observations will be carried out at the same time?

Using best evidence

In this situation providing effective care will be based on some research evidence in the use of thermometers. However, research has produced mixed results and the midwife may have to rely on the Trust policies and manufacturer's guidance in relation to the use of particular thermometers. Some questions that could arise are: How long should a thermometer be left in? What is the significance of breastfeeding? What is the significance of a painful wound? Is there any significance of her being anaemic? Is the result obtained in the normal range?

Professional and legal issues

Midwives must practise within a professional and legal framework. Questions that may arise from this scenario are: Is Jessica's use of her clinical judgement of timing of temperature taking appropriate? Are there any external Trust issues that are affecting her timing of taking the temperature? Is she using the correct equipment in the correct way? Does she refer the case to an appropriate professional and document her actions?

Team working

The midwife will not be working in isolation in the ward area. She will have other colleagues who will need to know about women who have abnormal temperatures so that they can be closely observed and monitored. Referral may need to be made to the medical team as well. Questions that may arise include: Where will the results of this

be recorded? Who should Julia inform? When should the temperature be repeated if at all? Who will need to be informed about this and how?

Clinical dexterity

The process of taking a temperature is covered above; however the equipment required will depend on the individual Trust and situation. The midwife will need to be familiar with all devices used for taking temperature in her locality. The skills required for taking temperatures involve communication and psychological care as well as the physical requirements of the task. Questions that may arise include: Is Julia familiar with the equipment available to use? If she is not how should she find out how to use it?

Models of care

Different trusts and ward areas organize care on shifts differently. In this situation Julia may be caring for Jessica as part of her case load as a student or as one of many on the ward. In a holistic woman-centred approach as indicated above the temperature will be taken as part of a whole person approach, considering all the aspects of Jessica's condition at the time. Questions that may arise include: If whole person care is being carried out how should Julia approach the issue of taking Jessica's temperature? How will the results affect the type of care given to an individual woman? What are the advantages of whole person care (rather than task orientated care) in this situation?

Safe environment

Hospital wards are renowned for being warm places. This may have an effect on the temperature of women and their babies. Furthermore, the use of plastic sheets to protect the beds or plastic covered duvets may increase the levels of heat. The use of electric fans or opening windows may provide a cooling atmosphere, but this must be balanced in relation to the effect of draughts on babies' temperature. Questions that could be asked include: Is the equipment being used safe for use with childbearing women? Is there any way the environmental temperature could be reduced in the postnatal area without causing risk to the baby? Are there different forms of mattress protection or bedding that could be used to reduce the risk of raising body temperatures?

Promotes health

Midwives have an opportunity with each encounter to promote health and wellbeing for the woman and her baby. In this situation Julia could use the opportunity to spend time with Jessica to find out about how she is feeling following the caesarean and carry out appropriate assessment of her whole wellbeing. Questions that arise include: How may Julia use this opportunity to promote health and wellbeing regarding temperature issues? How does Jessica assess temperature at home? What can Julia discuss in relation to learning about the baby's temperature and the environment? What are the safe sleeping recommendations for the temperature of the room where the baby sleeps?

Further scenarios

The following scenarios enable you to consider how specific situations influence the care the midwife provides. Use the jigsaw model to explore the issues raised in each scenario.

Scenario 1

Emily has given birth to Sarah an hour ago. It was a forceps birth and Sarah did not breathe spontaneously and required some oxygen on the resuscitaire. Emily is now having a wash and Clare the midwife is checking Sarah. She weighs 2.2 kg and feels cold to touch on her chest. Clare takes her temperature per axilla and notes it is 35.5 °C.

Practice point

In situations where the infant has required resuscitation it is important to ensure that they are kept warm and their needs considered in relation to those of the mother. In this situation it may have been more appropriate to continue skin-to-skin contact to ensure the baby retains her body warmth and commences feeding as soon as possible rather than meeting the hygiene needs of the mother.

Further questions specific to Scenario 1 include:

- What could be the significance of Sarah's birth weight?
- What equipment could be used to help warm Sarah?
- What other actions will Clare take to increase warmth?
- To whom should the information about the temperature be given?
- What further observations may be required?

Scenario 2

James is four days old following a normal birth. It has been noted that he has jaundice which is at a level requiring phototherapy treatment. Shauna, the midwife caring for him, locates a temperature chart and a thermometer.

Practice point

Though physiological jaundice is a common condition for newborn babies, special care still needs to be taken to ensure that there are no underlying pathological conditions. Treatment under light is the usual; however the baby is at risk of becoming dehydrated and hyperthermic.

Further questions specific to Scenario 2 include:

- How will the midwife ensure James remains hydrated?
- How often will the temperature need to be taken?
- What is the normal range of neonatal temperature and when should referral be made?
- What information will be given to the mother about James' temperature?
- What consideration should be made about environmental issues relating to James' care?

Conclusion

Taking a person's temperature is a skill required by midwives to ensure that observation can be made of wellbeing as body temperature control is important for good health. Consideration should be made of the types of equipment required and a practitioner should ensure knowledge of those that are available for use. Understanding of the reasons and value of the timing for taking temperature in the pregnancy continuum is important. Midwives should also be clear when a temperature is outside the normal range and the reasons for early referral to other practitioners.

Useful resources

NHS Direct information on how to take someone's temperature using different methods http://www.nhsdirect.nhs.uk/articles/article.aspx?articleId = 1065

http://en.wikipedia.org/wiki/Thermoregulation
http://en.wikipedia.org/wiki/Core_temperature

References

Baston H, Durward H 2001 Examination of the newborn: a practical guide. Routledge, London

Blows W T 2001 The biological basis of nursing: clinical observations. Routledge, London

Burroughs A, Leifer G 2001 Maternity nursing: an introductory text, 8th edn. WB Saunders, Philadelphia

Coad J 2006 Anatomy and physiology for midwives, 2nd edn. Mosby, Edinburgh

Department of Health 2004 Maternity Standard, National Service Framework for children, young people and maternity services. Department of Health, London

Guyton A C, Hall J 2007 Textbook of medical physiology, 11th edn. Elsevier, London

Johnson R, Taylor W 2006 Skills for midwifery practice, 2nd edn. Harcourt Health Sciences, Edinburgh

Mallik M, Hall C, Howard D 1998 Nursing knowledge and practice: a decision making approach. Baillière Tindall, London

McKinney E S, Ashwill J W, Murray S S et al 2000 Maternal-child nursing. WB Saunders, Philadelphia

National Institute for Health and Clinical Excellence (NICE) 2006 Routine postnatal care of women and their babies. NICE, London

National Institute for Health and Clinical Excellence (NICE) 2007 Intrapartum care. Care of healthy women and their babies during childbirth. NICE clinical guideline 55. NICE, London

National Institute for Health and Clinical Excellence (NICE) 2008 Antenatal care: routine care for the healthy pregnant woman. Clinical guideline 62. NICE, London

Nursing and Midwifery Council (NMC) 2004a Standards of proficiency for pre-registration midwifery education. NMC, London

Nursing and Midwifery Council (NMC) 2004b Midwives rules and standards. NMC, London

Nursing and Midwifery Council (NMC) 2008 The Code. Standards of conduct, performance and ethics. NMC, London

Purssell E 2007 Commentary on Farnell S, Maxwell L, Tan S et al 2005. Temperature measurement: comparison of non-invasive methods used in adult critical care. Journal of Clinical Nursing 16(1): 217–219

Stables D 2005 Physiology and childbearing with anatomy and related biosciences, 2nd edn. Baillière Tindall, Edinburgh

Chapter 6

Pulse and respiration

Introduction

The assessment of pulse and respiration within clinical practice is often referred to as 'doing the obs'. But this phrase, whilst in common usage, does sound very simple and fails to convey the significance of these basic, yet essential vital signs. The importance of these assessments is sometimes unrecognized and delay in acting upon abnormal results can severely compromise maternal and child health and wellbeing (Lewis 2007). Of the reported maternal deaths due to genital tract sepsis during the triennium 2003–2005, suboptimal care was identified in 70% of the cases, with a number of practitioners either not recognizing or failing to act upon signs and symptoms of infection such as raised pulse and respiratory rate (Lewis 2007).

This chapter will focus upon the assessment of pulse and respiration within midwifery practice, based upon a scenario. The background physiology of heart rate and respiration will be discussed and the physiology in relation to pregnancy will be explored. Using the framework within this book, the

procedure will be described and then the 'jigsaw model' will be used to consider relevant issues.

Trigger scenario

Consider the following scenario in relation to the measurement of a woman's pulse and respiratory rate.

Suzie was in advanced labour and coping well with regular contractions. Following a particularly strong contraction Suzie complained of feeling dizzy and light-headed. The midwife noted that her respiratory rate was rapid and encouraged Suzie to breathe more slowly by showing her how to breathe in through her nose and to blow gently out through her mouth. Suzie's pulse rate was raised but within normal limits.

What questions does this scenario raise? What information do you need to understand to enable you to interpret and make sense of this situation?

Your questions might include:

- Why did Suzie feel dizzy and light-headed?

- Could the strong contraction have contributed to this? Why?
- What is meant by the term 'respiratory rate'?
- How did the midwife know that Suzie's respiratory rate was rapid?
- What is a normal respiratory rate for an adult?
- Why did the midwife encourage Suzie to breathe more slowly?
- What is meant by the term 'pulse rate'?
- How did the midwife know that Suzie's pulse rate was raised?
- What are the normal limits for pulse rate for an adult?
- Does pregnancy and labour usually have an effect on the respiratory and pulse rate?

Background physiology of the pulse

During each cardiac cycle, as the left ventricle of the heart contracts, a wave of pressure is transmitted through the arterial system causing expansion and recoil of the arteries (Tortora 2005). This can be palpated, with the fingertips, in arteries lying close to the surface of the skin as a wave-like sensation called a pulse (Tortora & Grabowski 2003). The pulse can be palpated as being strongest in the arteries closer to the heart, becoming weaker as it passes through the arterioles and disappearing as it reaches the capillaries (Tortora & Grabowski 2003).

Activity

Access an anatomy text to remind you of the cardiac cycle and circulatory system.

Each pulse corresponds to a beat of the heart and when assessing the pulse, midwives should note the:

- rate
- rhythm and
- amplitude.

The heart rate is regulated by the sinoatrial (SA) node; the heart's internal pacemaker. The SA node sets a constant heart rate of approximately 100 beats per minute. During different circumstances, such as exercise, stress, haemorrhage or ill health, the body requires different volumes of blood flow to ensure that the oxygen and nutrient needs of the tissues and organs are met. To enable these requirements to be met a healthy heart is able to beat faster, or more slowly, under the influence of the autonomic nervous system, chemical regulation and a number of physical factors (Tortora & Grabowski 2003, Dougherty & Lister 2006).

In order to understand how the heart responds to these different circumstances, it is necessary to understand the terms heart rate, stroke volume and cardiac output.

- Heart rate is the number of beats of the heart over a period of 1 minute.
- Stroke volume is the amount of blood pumped out of the ventricle by each contraction of the heart.
- Cardiac output is the amount of blood pumped out of the heart in 1 minute.

So, cardiac output = stroke volume × heart rate.

The cardiovascular centre, in the medulla oblongata region of the brainstem, receives input from a range of sensory receptors; such as those monitoring movement, blood pressure and blood chemistry and from higher brain centres including the cerebral cortex, the limbic system and the hypothalamus. In response to this input, the cardiovascular centre then increases, or decreases, the frequency of nerve impulses to the heart via the cardiac accelerator nerves (sympathetic nervous system) and the vagus nerves (parasympathetic nerves) adjusting the heart rate. Increased sympathetic nerve stimulation leads to an increase in heart rate, whereas increased parasympathetic nerve stimulation leads to a decrease in heart rate (Tortora & Grabowski 2003, Tortora 2005, Dougherty & Lister 2006).

At rest, the normal pulse rate for an adolescent and an adult is between 60 and 100 beats per minute (bpm) (Dougherty & Lister 2006), whilst a newborn baby may have a pulse rate of over 120 beats per minute (Tortora & Grabowski 2003). During exercise, the body requires increased amounts of oxygen and nutrients so the heart must increase the rate at which it beats to increase cardiac output. Even before exercise occurs anticipatory changes may be noted as the limbic system generates anticipatory nerve impulses to the cardiovascular centre in the medulla, causing a rise in pulse rate. Once exercise begins the sensory receptors monitoring movement, blood chemistry and blood pressure send an increased frequency of nerve impulses to the cardiovascular centre and a rapid rise in pulse rate can be observed (Tortora & Grabowski 2003). If the circulating blood volume drops (hypovolaemia), for example during either an ante- or postpartum haemorrhage, the stroke volume declines and the blood pressure falls and in order to maintain cardiac output the heart must increase the rate at which it beats.

A number of chemicals, hormones and cations influence heart rate and the physiology of the cardiac muscle.

Hypoxia, acidosis and alkalosis all depress cardiac activity (Tortora & Grabowski 2003) whereas the hormones adrenaline and thyroxine increase heart rate. Several cations are essential for the initiation and maintenance of action potentials in nerve and muscle fibres and an imbalance of ions can quickly compromise cardiac output. Elevated blood levels of sodium and potassium decrease the heart rate whereas elevated levels of calcium increase the heart rate (Tortora & Grabowski 2003, Tortora 2005).

Physical factors which influence the resting heart rate include age, gender, body temperature and physical fitness (Tortora & Grabowski 2003). Adult females have been noted to have a slightly higher resting pulse than adult males (Tortora & Grabowski 2003).

Activity

Consider why the physical factors mentioned above may influence the resting heart rate.

Tachycardia is the term used to describe an elevated resting heart rate. In adults this is over 100 beats per minute. A tachycardia may be noted when there is an increased body temperature, for example in response to a postpartum infection. The raised body temperature causes the sinoatrial nerve to trigger more rapid contractions of the heart, increasing the heart rate (Tortora & Grabowski 2003).

Bradycardia is the term used to describe a resting heart rate of less than 60 beats per minute. A bradycardia may be noted when the body temperature is low, as a result of certain drugs or if the parasympathetic nervous system is stimulated. A bradycardia may also be observed in athletes who are physically and cardiovascularly well conditioned. As a result of increased stroke volume due to hypertrophy of the heart, the athlete's heart rate must be lower to maintain cardiac output.

The *pulse rhythm* is the sequence of beats (Dougherty & Lister 2006) and in a healthy individual this should be regular. Defects in the conduction system of the heart could cause uncoordinated contraction of the heart which could result in an irregular pulse.

The strength of a pulse reflects the elasticity of the arterial wall. If a woman is hypovolaemic, the greater the reduction in circulating blood volume, the more weak and thready the pulse will feel. A strong and bounding pulse may be an indication of infection (Trim 2004).

Activity

Find out what hypovolaemic means.

Background physiology of respiration

Respiration is the process of gas exchange within the body; oxygen is supplied to body cells to enable them to carry out their vital functions whilst carbon dioxide is removed. From a clinical perspective, the respiration rate is the number of breaths per minute.

When assessing respirations midwives should note the:

- rate
- rhythm and
- depth.

During respiration three events must occur; pulmonary ventilation, external respiration and internal respiration. Pulmonary ventilation, or breathing, is the movement of air into (inspiration) and out of (expiration) the lungs. The pressure changes within the lungs and thoracic cavity during inspiration and expiration result in the flow of gases to equalize pressure (Tortora & Grabowski 2003, Richardson 2006). Just before inspiration, the air pressure inside the lungs is equal to the pressure in the atmosphere so, for air to move into the lungs, the pressure inside the lungs must become lower than atmospheric pressure. This is achieved by increasing the volume of the lungs. As the lungs are tightly adherent to the diaphragm and thoracic wall, an increase in the volume of the thoracic cavity will result in an increase in the volume of the lungs. The volume of the thoracic cavity increases due to contraction of the dome-shaped diaphragm and the external intercostal muscles. Contraction of the diaphragm makes the diaphragm flatten, increasing the vertical dimension of the thoracic cavity (Tortora and Grabowski 2003, Richardson 2006). This is accompanied with contraction of the muscles lying between the ribs, the external intercostal muscles. This causes the rib cage to rise up and move outwards, increasing the front to back and side to side dimensions of the thoracic cavity (Tortora & Grabowski 2003, Dougherty & Lister 2004, Tortora 2005). The air in the lungs now has a larger area to fill and so the pressure falls and air flows into the lungs until the pressure in the lungs (intrapulmonary pressure) equals the atmospheric pressure.

Expiration occurs as the inspiratory muscles relax. The diaphragm moves upwards, returning to its dome shape. The external intercostal muscles return to their resting position causing the rib cage to descend and the volume of the thoracic cavity, and hence the lungs, decreases. This process is aided by the elastic recoil properties of the lungs. As the volume of the lungs decreases, the pressure inside the lungs increases and as this pressure is now greater than atmospheric pressure, air must flow out of the lungs to equalize pressure. The degree to which the lungs are able to stretch and recoil and the thorax is able to expand and relax during inspiration and expiration is called lung compliance.

External respiration is the exchange of gases between the air spaces of the lungs and the pulmonary capillary blood. The blood loses carbon dioxide and gains oxygen. The exchange of carbon dioxide and oxygen between the capillaries and tissue cells is called internal respiration (Tortora 2005).
The blood loses oxygen and gains carbon dioxide.

Activity

Access an anatomy and physiology text book and revise the anatomical structures and physiology of respiration.

Control of respiration

The rhythm of normal, quiet breathing is set by the respiratory control centre, located in the medulla oblongata of the brainstem and respiration usually occurs without conscious effort. The inspiratory area of the respiratory control centre contains neurones responsible for inspiration and expiration and it is the nervous impulses generated within this area which control the rhythm of breathing.
A respiratory cycle, that is inspiration

followed by expiration, is usually five seconds, giving a normal respiratory rate for an adult of approximately 12 breaths per minute.

This basic rhythm would suffice if individuals were to remain at rest, however, in order to meet the changing demands of the body, there are a number of nervous and chemical factors which affect the respiratory centre altering the rate and depth of respiration.

Anticipation of activity, emotion, pain and fear can all cause stimulation of the limbic system which results in excitatory input to the inspiratory area, increasing the rate and depth of breathing (Tortora 2005). This increase is referred to as tachypnoea. An increase in body temperature increases the rate of respiration by about seven breaths per minute for every one degree raise in body temperature as the body tries to regulate its temperature and cool down (Dougherty & Lister 2004) whereas a decrease in body temperature is accompanied by a decrease in respiratory rate, bradypnoea (Tortora & Grabowski 2003, Tortora 2005). Opiate narcotics can also cause a decrease in respiratory rate as the action of the respiratory centre within the medulla oblongata is depressed (Dougherty & Lister 2004) whilst stimulants such as caffeine and amphetamines can cause tachypnoea (Richardson 2003).

The function of the respiratory system is to maintain the correct levels of oxygen and carbon dioxide in the blood and body fluids to meet the demands of the body. If there are changes to these levels sensory neurones called chemoreceptors are stimulated. If there is even just a slight increase in the level of carbon dioxide in the blood the chemoreceptors send nervous impulses to the brain which causes the inspiratory area to become more active, increasing the rate of respiration. The body expels more carbon dioxide, the carbon dioxide level is lowered back to normal levels and the respiratory rate returns to normal. Similarly, if the level of carbon dioxide in the blood is lower than normal the chemoreceptors and the neurones in the inspiratory area are not stimulated and the rate of respiration slows down until the level of carbon dioxide in the blood returns to normal (Tortora 2005).

Physiology in relation to pregnancy

Boxes 6.1 and 6.2 illustrate the physiological effects in relation to pregnancy.

Activity

Find out what hyperventilation means.

National guidance

The National Service Framework for Children, Young People and Maternity Services (Department of Health 2004) stipulates the provision of individualized, woman-centred care which entails using appropriate observations for the appropriate situation. Further, there is the requirement for midwives to be able to recognize when a woman needs

---

Box 6.1 Physiological effects on pulse in relation to pregnancy

Antenatal period

What happens Heart rate rises (approx. 20%), about 15 beats per min and stroke volume increases

Why Increased demands of maternal organs and developing fetus

What happens Heart size increases by approx 12%

Why Cardiac muscle hypertrophy stimulated by oestrogen and increased filling.

Intrapartum

What happens Heart rate increases

Why Strenuous nature of labour and birth and muscular activity of uterus

What happens Increase in cardiac output

Why Circulating volume increases as 300–500 ml of blood enter the circulation during contractions. Also exacerbated by pain, anxiety and fear.

Postnatal

What happens Circulating volume and cardiac output fall with stroke volume remaining high leading to reduction in heart rate

Why Less pressure as reduction in pressure from increased weight load. Hypertrophy of the ventricles.

Coad 2006

referral to other practitioners within the multiprofessional team.

There is no specific guidance relating to pulse and respiration in the NICE guidelines for antenatal care (NICE 2008). In the NICE intrapartum guideline (NICE 2007) a woman's pulse should be taken as an observation when labour is suspected and should be observed when listening to the fetal heart, to ensure there is differentiation between the two. The pulse should be taken hourly in the first and second stages of labour and hourly in the second stage of labour and immediately following birth.

Box 6.2 Physiological effects on respiration in relation to pregnancy

Antenatal period

What happens Early in pregnancy, pregnancy hormones cause increase in the respiratory excursion of the diaphragm, increased flaring of the lower ribs and broadening of the chest. This means during respiration the volume of a normal breath (tidal volume) increases and during expiration the chest wall moves further inwards resulting in a decrease in the residual volume in the lungs.

By the end of pregnancy up to 20% more oxygen is consumed than in the non-pregnant state. The respiratory rate remains unchanged

Why It enables the increased metabolic demands of the mother and fetus to be met, as well as to compensate for the increasing size and volume of the uterus

It is these changes which increase the efficiency of alveolar gas exchange during pregnancy, whilst the rate of respiration remains unchanged.

Intrapartum period

What happens Labour and birth lead to increase of respiratory rate and depth

Why Partly in response to increased muscular work which raises the metabolic rate and oxygen consumption and partly in response to the effects of pain, anxiety and drugs

What happens Women may experience dizziness and tingling in the fingers and toes. In early labour, this may be transient and short lasting, however it may cause respiratory alkalosis and increased blood pH

Why Due to hyperventilation as a result of pain and anxiety

What happens During established labour hyperventilation may be exacerbated. The birth partner or midwife can support her by guiding her to consciously slow down her breathing rate following contractions.

Postnatal period

What happens In normal circumstances respiration rates will rapidly return to normal levels following birth. However it is appropriate to maintain observations, especially postoperatively

Why Affecting the rate may be fatigue, anaemia, haemorrhage, pain or anxiety.

Coad 2006

The NICE guidelines for postnatal care (2006) state that midwives should ask at each postnatal examination about a woman's health and should assess appropriately. This indicates the use of observations of pulse and respirations only when thought to be clinically required.

Professional guidelines

To practise midwifery in the United Kingdom, midwives must abide by the rules, standards and codes of the Nursing and Midwifery Council. The activities of a midwife as described in *Midwives rules and standards* include 'recognize the warning signs of abnormality in the mother or infant' (NMC 2004a:37). The midwife must therefore use her clinical observational skills to fulfil her role. Rule 6 stipulates that it is a midwife's responsibility to refer deviations from normal in the woman or baby to an appropriate health professional (page 16). The Guidelines for Records and record keeping (NMC 2005) require professionals to maintain records that 'provide clear evidence of care planned, the decisions made, the care delivered and the information shared' (page 8) and this clearly includes all clinical observations.

The assessment of pulse and respiratory rate

Pulse

When assessing a woman's pulse, the practitioner should note the rate, rhythm and strength of the pulse. It is important to remember that even if a woman's vital signs are being continuously monitored by automated equipment it is essential to still manually assess the rhythm and strength of the pulse, as the equipment will only give a reading of the pulse rate. The ability to detect changes in the rhythm and strength of the pulse is a skill which takes time to develop but it is valuable for safe practice.

To assess the pulse it is necessary to gently press the artery against a firm structure such as a bone. The site most commonly used in adults is the radial artery which is located in the inner aspect of the wrist at the base of the thumb. Other sites include the temporal artery and the carotid, brachial, popliteal, femoral, posterior tibial and dorsalis pedis arteries. To assess the pulse rate (heart rate) of a neonate, it is usual to auscultate the heart rate by placing a stethoscope directly over the heart. Alternatively, the pulse may be felt at the base of the umbilicus immediately following birth.

Activity

Access the Standards of proficiency for pre-registration midwifery education (NMC 2004b) and The Code. Standards of conduct, performance and ethics (NMC 2008). Consider which standards are relevant to the issue of observing pulse and respirations.

Activity

Try and locate your own pulse on your wrist, neck, groin, behind your knee and your foot. Consider when you may need to assess pulse rates at these sites, if ever, in pregnant women.

Respiratory rate

The normal rate of respiration for an adult at rest is between 14 and 18 breaths per minute, with the ratio of pulse rate to respiration rate being approximately 5 to 1 (Dougherty & Lister 2004). Newborn infants' rate of respiration is much faster than this, at between 30 and 80 breaths per minute. The most usual time to assess a woman's rate is following taking her pulse and whilst still holding her wrist, so that she does not change her pattern of breathing while being observed.

The volume of air moving in and out with each respiration is referred to as the depth of respiration (Dougherty & Lister 2004). Normal respiration is almost silent, regular and effortless.

Activity

Find out what is meant by dyspnoea. What signs may a woman show that she is making extra respiratory effort?

To assess the respiratory rate, depth and pattern of a neonate, place the flats of the fingers over the chest for 1 minute.

Equipment for pulse and respiration

In usual circumstances all that are required will be a watch or clock with a second hand. However, midwives should be aware of how to use any electronic methods of measuring rates in their places of work.

1. The midwife discusses the procedure with the woman enabling her to understand its relevance to her care and give consent

Though the taking of a pulse may be very familiar to most women it is important to explain any procedure and request consent prior to touching the woman. Some women may feel

---

Box 6.3 Procedure for checking pulse and respiration

- **Consult the client's plan of care**

  Rationale To ensure that the client's condition is monitored effectively. To establish the frequency of observations required for each individual. The client should be sufficiently involved in her care that she is expecting to have her pulse measured

- **Gain verbal consent from the client**

  Rationale Consent for this procedure is often implied by an outstretched arm. However, it is courteous to ask before attempting to take a pulse, and to talk to women who appear to be asleep

- **Locate the required equipment (a watch or clock with a second hand)**

  Rationale To ensure preparation and accuracy for the observation

- **Wash hands thoroughly**

  Rationale To reduce the risk of cross infection

- **Give explanation of procedure if first time**

  Rationale To ensure the woman understands what is intended

continued

Box 6.3 continued

- **Woman should be comfortably sitting or lying on side**
  Rationale To avoid vena-caval compression
- **The second and third fingers should be placed over the selected artery, gently pressing against the bone to feel for the pulse**
  Rationale To avoid using the thumb and forefinger which have a pulse of their own and to avoid mistaking this for the woman's pulse. To avoid occluding the artery by too much pressure
- **The pulse should then be counted for 60 seconds**
  Rationale To allow sufficient time to detect any irregularities of rate, rhythm or character
- **The strength of the pulse should be assessed. It may be described as normal, weak, 'thready' or bounding**
  Rationale To recognize any abnormalities
- **Whilst still holding the woman's wrist following palpation of the radial artery, observe the respiratory rate, regularity and effort for 1 minute**

- *Rationale* To recognize any abnormalities
- **It may be appropriate to hold her wrist over her chest**
  Rationale To facilitate detection of each breath as the woman inspires and expires
- **Following the procedure ensure the woman is comfortable**
  Rationale To maintain her dignity and comfort
- **Inform the woman of the result and its significance**
  Rationale To ensure she is involved in her care
- **Wash the hands thoroughly again**
  Rationale To prevent cross infection
- **Record the results on the appropriate chart and any abnormalities in the notes**
  Rationale To ensure continuity, completeness and compliance with professional standards
- **Report any abnormalities to the appropriate person (NMC 2004)**
  Rationale To ensure appropriate care is given and the rules of practice complied with.

uncomfortable if too much pressure is exerted on the wrist. The practitioner can ascertain if the woman is familiar with the procedure through simple questioning, avoiding inappropriately lengthy explanations. Questions are likely to concern whether the pulse is normal. It is therefore important to be familiar with normal testing values for women and babies. The implications

of abnormal values need careful explanation.

2. The observation is made at the appropriate time according to the woman's plan of care

Where the pulse and respiration are observed as part of an individual plan of care this should he clearly documented and evaluated. Women should be assessed individually for their needs but the general guidance is in Box 6.4.

3. The observation is made using the correct technique

The midwife should be aware of the different methods of counting a pulse or respiration and how to do so. Counting for the appropriate length of

time is also important, as well as recognizing the strength. (See Box 6.3.)

4. The woman is supported during the observation and her reaction observed

Some women may find pressure on the wrist uncomfortable if pressed too hard or for too long. It is wise

---

Box 6.4 Indications for assessment of the pulse and respiration during the antenatal period, labour, birth, puerperium and neonatal period

Antenatal period

Heart rate To determine a baseline rate against which changes in pulse rate can be monitored. These changes may be an indication of fear, pain or occur as a result of infection or the administration of medication

Respiratory rate To determine a baseline rate against which changes in respiration can be monitored. These changes may be an indication of fear, pain or occur as a result of infection. The baseline rate should also be assessed prior to administration of prescribed opiate medication such as pethidine or if drug misuse is suspected.

Intrapartum period

Heart rate The maternal pulse rate should be palpated at the same time as the fetal heart is auscultated to ensure that the midwife is able to differentiate between fetal heart and maternal heart rate (Royal College of Obstetricians & Gynaecologists 2001) (NICE 2007)

Respiratory rate Awareness is required that opioid analgesia may affect the respiratory centre of the brain (BNF 2007).

  Included as an assessment of wellbeing for the third stage of labour (NICE 2007).

Postnatal period

Heart rate Following birth as part of the assessment of the physical wellbeing of the mother. This is important as an elevated pulse rate could be an early indication of postpartum haemorrhage or haematoma formation. The pulse should be assessed again prior to the attending midwife leaving the home or transfer of the woman from the delivery suite to the postnatal area and compared against the baseline to detect abnormalities.

  Following caesarean section it is recommended that the pulse rate and rhythm, in addition to blood pressure, respiratory rate, oxygen saturations, pain and sedation levels are monitored every 5 minutes for the first 30 minutes and then, if the woman is stable, half hourly for the first 2 hours (NICE 2004).

Prior to, during, and following, a blood transfusion when an elevated pulse rate may indicate sepsis, circulatory overload or febrile reactions (Dougherty & Lister 2004).

Respiratory rate Following birth as part of the assessment of the physical wellbeing of the mother.

Following caesarean section it is recommended that respiratory rate is one of the vital signs monitored every 5 minutes for the first 30 minutes and then, if the woman is stable, half-hourly for the first 2 hours (NICE 2004).

Neonatal period

Heart rate Assessment of the neonate's heart rate following birth to determine successful transition to neonatal life

Respiratory rate The baby's respirations should be assessed 1 minute after birth and, if within normal limits, then again at 5 minutes following birth to assess successful transition to extrauterine life. If the baby has been exposed to meconium liquor or there is suspected meconium inhalation during birth regular assessment of the respirations should be undertaken (NCCWCH 2007)

Heart rate and respiration rate should be observed following prolonged pre-labour rupture of membranes (more than 24 hours) at 1 hour, 2 hours and then 2-hourly for 10 hours (NICE 2007).

---

not to take a pulse on the arm where an intravenous infusion or needle is sited.

5. The woman is made comfortable after the measurement

The comfort of the woman should not be compromised if her arm is kept resting on the chair, bed or lap during this procedure.

6. The woman is informed of the result

If the result is in the normal range this should be indicated to the woman. If results are outside the normal range

the significance of this should be explained to her carefully, especially in relation to her baby, as it may cause her anxiety.

7. If the result is outside normal parameters it is reported to an appropriate member of the team

As indicated above, the midwife should understand the significance of the ranges of pulse and respiration rates in pregnant and postnatal women. If the values fall outside what is regarded as normal she should inform a registered practitioner and other relevant members of the midwifery team of her findings.

8. An accurate and legible record is made of the observation

Readings must be recorded on the appropriate documentation and in black ink. Where any action was taken as a result of the observation this should also be documented and a plan of care developed.

Reflection on trigger scenario

Reconsider the trigger scenario at the start of the chapter:

Suzie was in advanced labour and coping well with regular contractions. Following a particularly strong contraction Suzie complained of feeling dizzy and light-headed. The midwife noted that her respiratory rate was rapid and encouraged Suzie to breathe more slowly by showing her how to breathe in through her nose and to blow gently out through her mouth. Suzie's pulse rate was raised but within normal limits.

In the trigger scenario it is reported that Suzie had a rapid respiratory rate and slightly elevated pulse rate following a particularly strong contraction. She was experiencing dizziness and feeling light-headed; both symptoms of hyperventilation. Suzie's midwife noted these abnormalities, but having developed knowledge of the underpinning physiology was able to apply theoretical knowledge to midwifery practice and instruct Suzie to consciously slow down her respiratory rate, relieving Suzie's unpleasant symptoms.

Effective communication

As Suzie is in advanced labour, the periods between contractions when she will be able to focus upon the midwife's explanation will be limited so the midwife must carefully consider her use of language and make explanations succinct. It may be helpful to consider how you would explain this situation to a woman in this situation. Questions that may arise include: How should a midwife speak to a woman in strong labour? What other ways may the midwife communicate with Suzie?

Woman-centred care

Whole person care of Suzie will involve complete assessment of why she is experiencing her symptoms. Further, to enhance Suzie's continuing care her midwife should explain why she was experiencing these unpleasant symptoms and how she can control her breathing pattern to minimize the risk of recurrence. The midwife should also explain the importance of ongoing assessment of her health and wellbeing through monitoring of her vital signs including pulse and respirations. By engaging Suzie in discussion about these assessments she is then able to make informed consent regarding ongoing care and observation. Questions that may arise include: How can the midwife ensure the woman's choices are being met during assessment of her wellbeing?

Using best evidence

There is little research evidence regarding the efficacy of the duration of assessment of pulse and respirations. Historically these have been counted for 15 seconds and then multiplied by 4 to give the rate per minute. However, this short duration of assessment offers little opportunity to detect an abnormal rhythm and so it is recommended that the pulse and respirations are counted for at least 30 seconds, but preferably 60 seconds. If an abnormality is detected then the pulse and respirations should be counted for 60 seconds. Some questions that could arise include: Is the use of a watch or clock accurate? Is any mechanical equipment used reliable?

Professional and legal

Midwives must practise within a professional and legal framework. With regard to the charting of vital signs, each Trust may have different observation charts and local guidance; however accurate record keeping is required to meet the NMC guidance and a failure to do so falls below the standard required of midwifery practitioners and is unacceptable. Questions that may arise from this scenario include: Is the midwife following current guidelines in her assessment of Suzie's pulse and respirations? Is she using the correct equipment in the correct way? Is her documentation of the results accurate?

Team working

Once the midwife has assessed and recorded Suzie's vital signs she must then consider if the findings fall within the normal range for the individual client (NMC 2004a, NMC 2005). If an abnormality is detected, the midwife must refer to other members of the team, as appropriate (NMC 2004a). This will necessitate working with other midwives as well as a range of other professionals such as obstetricians and paediatricians. Questions that arise include: How should other professionals be informed? When should they be informed? Where should referral be documented? What should the midwife

do if a practitioner does not respond to her referral?

Clinical dexterity

Assessment of Suzie's pulse and respirations during advanced labour requires the midwife to have a degree of clinical dexterity. As a coping strategy during labour Suzie may be moving around, rocking or swaying. The midwife needs to have developed her basic skills of assessing pulse and respirations to be able to apply them in this situation and novice practitioners must capitalize upon opportunities to develop these skills so that they are able to apply them in more complex situations. Questions that arise include: Is the midwife familiar with the equipment available for use? If she is not how should she find out how to use it? What should she do if she is finding it difficult to feel the radial pulse? When is the best time to make such observation of the neonate?

Safe environment

To safely assess pulse and respirations requires somewhere to wash your hands and a watch or clock with a second hand. Failure to attend to infection control issues may compromise Suzie's safety. Reliance upon wall mounted clocks may lead to limiting Suzie's freedom of movement or mobility which is unacceptable. Questions that may arise include: Is the watch kept where it will not scratch either the mother or her newborn baby? What measures can be taken to reduce the risk of cross infection between women?

Promotes health

The assessment of pulse and respiration is a non-invasive procedure which should not pose any challenges to either maternal or neonatal health. Questions that may arise include: How may the midwife use this opportunity to promote maternal health and wellbeing regarding the observations made? What information could you give new parents about the baby's breathing patterns?

Further scenarios

The following scenarios enable you to consider how specific situations influence the care the midwife provides. Use the jigsaw model to explore the issues raised in each scenario.

Scenario 1

At an antenatal appointment Emily, who is 30 weeks pregnant with her first baby, complains of feeling breathless and dizzy. Marian, her midwife, asks if this has been recent and Emily replies it has only been in the past two weeks. Marian asks if she can take Emily's pulse.

Practice point

In the second trimester of pregnancy some women may show symptoms of anaemia. This may lead to women feeling breathless and dizzy as the body requires more iron. The definitive diagnosis is usually through testing of the blood for iron levels. However, there may be alternative reasons for her symptoms.

Further questions might include:

- What may counting her pulse show?
- Why does Marian ask Emily if this is recent?
- What is the alternative diagnosis for these symptoms?
- What other observations may she make on Emily to aid in her diagnosis?
- What may she expect to find on taking her pulse and why?

- If the pulse rate is significantly abnormal what will she do now?
- Where will she document her findings?

Scenario 2

Pippa has had a normal birth three days ago. Fiona visits her at home and thinks she is looking very pale. She asks is she can take her pulse, and finds it is very fast and her breathing fast. Fiona asks if she has a heavy blood loss and Pippa says 'yes'.

Practice point

Following the third stage of labour occasionally a small part of the placenta or membranes may remain in the uterus. The midwife should always be alert to this potential problem as it could lead to infection or secondary postpartum haemorrhage.

Further questions might include:

- Why might Fiona be looking pale?
- What are the reasons for her pulse and respirations being fast?
- What other observations may Fiona carry out to assess Pippa's wellbeing?
- Where will she record her observations?
- Whom will she advise of her observations?
- What actions may need to be taken?

Conclusion

Assessment of pulse and respirations are essential skills for midwifery practitioners to develop to enable monitoring of health and wellbeing as well as identifying abnormalities which could indicate a number of complications. Developing dexterity in these skills and the knowledge required to underpin interpretation of the findings and to plan care requires practice and attention to detail.

Useful resources

Dougherty L, Lister S 2004 The Royal Marsden Hospital manual of clinical nursing procedures, 6th edn. Blackwell Publishing, Oxford. Comment: This book offers up-to-date, evidence-based, information regarding both basic and more complex nursing procedures, many of which are transferable to midwifery practice.

Vital signs

http://www.rwjuh.edu/health_information/adult_nontrauma_vital.html

References

British National Formulary (BNF) Joint Formulary Committee 2007 54th edn. British Medical Association and Royal Pharmaceutical Society of Great Britain, London

Coad J 2006 Anatomy and physiology for midwives. Elsevier Limited, Edinburgh

Department of Health 2004 Maternity Standard, National Service Framework for children, young people and maternity services. Department of Health, London

Dougherty L, Lister S 2006 The Royal Marsden Hospital manual of clinical nursing procedures, 6th edn. Blackwell Publishing, Oxford

Lewis G (ed) 2007 Confidential enquiry into maternal and child health. Saving mothers' lives: 2003–2005. The seventh report on confidential enquirires into maternal deaths in the United Kingdom. CEMACH, London

National Institute for Health and Clinical Excellence (NICE) 2003 Antenatal care: routine care for the healthy pregnant woman. Clinical guideline 6. NICE, London

National Institute for Health and Clinical Excellence (NICE) 2004 National Collaborating Centre for Women's and Children's Health Caesarean section. RCOG Press, London

National Institute for Health and Clinical Excellence (NICE) 2006 Routine postnatal care of women and their babies. NICE, London

National Institute for Health and Clinical Excellence (NICE) 2007 Intrapartum care. Care of healthy women and their babies during childbirth. NICE clinical guideline 55. NICE, London

Nursing and Midwifery Council (NMC) 2004a Midwives rules and standards. NMC, London

Nursing and Midwifery Council (NMC) 2004b Standards of proficiency for pre-registration midwifery education. NMC, London

Nursing and Midwifery Council (NMC) 2005 Records and record keeping. NMC, London

Nursing and Midwifery Council (NMC) 2008 The Code. Standards of conduct, performance and ethics for nurses and midwives. NMC, London

Richardson M 2003 Physiology for practice: the mechanisms controlling respiration. Nursing Times 99(48)

Richardson M 2006 The respiratory system – Part 4: breathing. Nursing Times 102(26)

Royal College of Obstetricians and Gynaecologists 2001 The use of electronic fetal monitoring. The use and interpretation of cardiotocography in intrapartum fetal surveillance. Evidence based clinical guideline number 8. RCOG Press, London

Tortora G J 2005 Principles of human anatomy, 10th edn. Wiley, New York

Tortora G J, Grabowski S R 2003 Principles of anatomy and physiology, 10th edn. Wiley, New York

Trim J 2004 Performing a comprehensive physiological assessment. Nursing Times 100(50): 38–42

Chapter 7

Collection of specimens

Introduction

This chapter describes the principles and procedures for collecting a range of specimens, as part of the process of assessing the wellbeing of the mother and baby. The purpose of the collection of these specimens is to carry out tests or analysis in order to diagnose and treat any deviations from health. The specimens may be swabs from the mother or baby, or samples of body fluids and wastes. The midwife needs to know why and how these tests are carried out, in what circumstances such specimens might be required, and what to do with the information received in terms of ongoing care planning. Urine and blood testing are dealt with in separate chapters.

Trigger scenario

Consider the following scenario and what information you need to know to help you understand the situation in relation to specimen collection.

Sascha was 32 weeks pregnant with her second baby, and had had Group B Streptococcus infection in her first pregnancy. She came into the delivery suite for a high vaginal swab. 'Why do I have to have this swab taken again?' Sascha asks. 'I had antibiotics last time, and the baby was okay. I really don't like having this done.'

What do you need to know in order to interpret this situation?

Reflecting on this scenario you may ask yourself the following:

- What is Group B *Streptococcus* (GBS) infection?
- Why is Sascha having a high vaginal swab taken in this pregnancy?
- What is the procedure?
- Why might Sascha find it unpleasant?
- How are swabs used to detect infection or disease?
- How can the midwife ensure Sascha is not distressed by the procedure?

Background

When a midwife is requested to take a specimen from a mother and baby, it is usually when there is suspicion of infection, or as part of screening when women or babies have identified risk factors. It involves collecting material from the suspected source of the infection such as urine, or wound exudate collected on a swab. Culturing and identifying the micro-organism obtained by the swab or specimen allows for specific antibiotics to be prescribed for that particular micro-organism in order to treat and eradicate the infection (Johnson & Taylor 2006).

Neonatal sepsis

Neonatal infection has been described as infection which occurs during the first four weeks of life (HPA 2005). It may be superficial, such as conjunctivitis or skin infections, or deep infection, such as pneumonia or meningitis (HPA 2005). Neonatal infection is further subdivided into *early onset* infection, which occurs in the first 48 hours of life and is usually caused by infection ascending from the maternal genital tract, or *late onset*, which occurs after the first 48 hours of life where organisms may be acquired from the external environment (HPA 2005).

Risk factors to the development of neonatal sepsis include: congenital abnormalities; low birth weight; pre-term birth; prolonged rupture of the membranes; maternal fever; prolonged labour or birth trauma; respiratory distress syndrome; pre-eclampsia; babies of mothers who have previously had a baby affected by GBS.

Obtaining specimens

Swabs

Swabs should ideally be taken before antibiotic therapy has been commenced (Mallik et al 2004). There are specific swabs for particular purposes depending on the organism to be tested for, although for the majority of cases a dry swab plunged and sealed into a normal transport medium will suffice (Johnson & Taylor 2006). The dry swab should be fully coated in the fluid sampled by gentle rotation at the site of collection. All swabs should be clearly labelled with the site of sampling. So if it is the umbilicus, this should be stated, and if it is the ear or eye, which ear or eye should also be clearly stated. Samples should also be labelled with the time of collection as well as the date and patient identification.

Activity

Find out what transport media are required when testing for *Chlamydia* and *Trichomonas*.

Vaginal swabs

The kinds of specimens that might be taken include high vaginal and low vaginal swabs, to test for Group B *Streptococcus* or for sexually transmitted infections. Group B *Streptococcus* has been found to be the most frequent cause of early onset infection in newborn babies (RCOG 2003). Therefore, in women classed to be at risk of GBS, diagnosis can allow doctors to attempt to prevent the infection of the newborn.

Swabs are taken from the vagina (see procedure in Box 7.1 below), either a high vaginal swab taken from the top of the vagina using a speculum (McKay-Moffat & Lee 2006), or a low vaginal swab taken from inside the introitus. Low vaginal swabs may detect the presence of infection in lochia, suggestive of intrauterine infection, for example.

Eye, ear, nasal and umbilical swabs

Swabs taken from these areas are used to detect colonization by micro-organisms that can cause infection and illness, either in mother (except for umbilical swabs) or baby.

Eye swab: the woman should be sitting up with the head supported; the baby should be held with its head supported, preferably by its mother or father. The lower eyelid is pulled down very gently, and the swab held parallel to the cornea to avoid injury (especially if the baby moves), and then moved gently against the conjunctiva of the lower eyelid (Johnson & Taylor 2006). The swab is then placed in the transport medium, sealed, labelled and sent via the appropriate route to the laboratory. Separate swabs should be taken from each eye.

Ear swab: seat the woman with her head tilted to the unaffected side; the baby should be firmly held with the unaffected ear against its parent's chest, with the head tilting upwards slightly (Johnson & Taylor 2006). The swab is placed gently into the outer ear and rotated. Some sources recommend straightening the external canal by gently pulling the pinna upwards and backwards, but care should be taken not to insert the swab too deeply in this case as there is a risk of damage to the eardrum. As with the eye, if both ears are to be swabbed, separate swabs should be taken from each ear.

Nose swab: seat the woman with her head tilted back; the baby can be held or laid supine. The swab should be moistened with sterile water, then inserted gently into the nose, directed towards the front of the nose and rotated (Johnson & Taylor 2006).

Throat swab: ask the woman to tilt her head backwards and stick out her tongue. Wearing gloves, depress the middle of the tongue with a disposable tongue depressor (like a large lollipop stick) and rub the tip of the dry swab around the tonsil area, taking care not to touch the lips or teeth (Timby 2005). Avoid the back of the throat as touching this stimulates the gag reflex and may make her vomit.

Umbilical swab: the baby should be held or positioned to provide access to the umbilicus, and clothing/nappy should be removed. As with other swabs, the tip should be rotated around the surface of the umbilicus and then the specimen labelled with the baby's information before being sent to the laboratory.

Activity

Identify the appropriate forms used where you work for sending specimens for the following examination: histology, virology, chemical pathology, microbiology.

Wound swabs

Wound infection can prevent or slow down wound healing. The kinds of wounds midwives will see include vaginal, vulval and perineal lacerations or tears, which may have been sutured, and postoperative wounds, typically from a caesarean section. Wound sampling can provide key biological information which, if interpreted in conjunction with the overall clinical picture, can inform optimal care management and planning (Gilchrist 2000). Midwives will generally undertake superficial wound sampling, from wounds where there are obvious signs of infection or where drains have been removed.

Placental specimens

Placental swabs

The swab should be moved across the surface of the placenta in a zigzag direction (Johnson & Taylor 2006). The swab should be labelled appropriately and the placenta disposed of in the usual manner.

Placental histology

Histological examination of the placenta may be indicated in certain clinical situations, requiring that the whole placenta or a portion of it be sent to the laboratory. This might be the case following a multiple birth, for example, to determine whether the infants are monozygous or dizygous or if there are any anomalies. It might also be necessary in preterm births, or following a stillbirth (Medforth et al 2006). In some cases it might also be a requirement to send the placenta itself where infection is suspected. Other indications include the birth of infants with congenital abnormalities, a two-vessel umbilical cord, and placental abruption.

The placenta (or segment) should be placed in a suitable specimen container, labelled with the correct details, and sent to the laboratory. Placentas are usually sent in large bucket-like containers with close-fitting lids. These are often supplied 'dry' (i.e. empty), for immediate transport to the laboratory during laboratory hours, or 'wet', partially filled with a formaldehyde fluid, for when the sample cannot be immediately sent, for example during the night. Care should be taken not to spill the preserving fluid when placing the placenta in the container. Universal precautions should be followed when handling placental specimens, and all waste should be disposed of appropriately.

Sputum sample

Sputum samples may be taken to detect certain contagious diseases; in particular TB in women who have not been immunized against the disease. Ask the woman to rinse her mouth with water first, to avoid contamination of the sample. Then ask her to expectorate into a sputum pot, which is sealed, labelled and sent to the laboratory according to Trust policy. Ensure you wear gloves for the procedure.

Stool sample

Stool samples may be screened for a variety of infectious diseases, including gastrointestinal diseases which may be highly contagious. A standard stool specimen pot is used, which contains a 'scoop' within the lid to assist in collecting the sample. If the woman is in hospital, you can offer a disposable bedpan to place on the toilet for stool collection: a small sample only is necessary. Advice about hygiene is important, and again, as a member of staff you should wear gloves and an apron and ensure you have washed your hands thoroughly following the procedure.

Activity

Locate the sample containers in your clinical area. Identify those used for urine, sputum, stool and other samples, and note the different kinds of containers. Some contain reagents necessary for detection of certain substances or micro-organisms. Identify the different swabs used, and note which swabs and specimen containers are used for which test or in which circumstances.

National guidance

The RCOG Guideline on prevention of neonatal Group B *Streptococcus* infection (RCOG 2003), suggests that women who have identified Group B *Streptococcus* infection in pregnancy should be offered prophylactic antibiotics in labour. It describes when and why women should be tested for this infection in pregnancy and labour.

Activity

Access the RCOG Guideline No 36 at http://www.rcog.org. uk/resources/Public/pdf/GroupB_strep_no36.pdf, and make a list of the recommendations for testing of women for Group B *Streptococcus* in pregnancy.

The HPA (2005) have published a standard operating procedure for investigation of infection screen swabs from the neonate.

Activity

Access the HPA guidance at:

www.hpa-standardmethods.org. uk/documents/bsop/pdf/bsop23.pdf

List the organisms which commonly cause neonatal infection, and how these are treated. Evaluate the role of the midwife in the monitoring and treatment of neonatal infection in the light of these guidelines.

Professional guidelines

Midwives who practise in the United Kingdom must work within the professional regulatory framework of the Nursing and Midwifery Council (NMC).

Activity

Access the Standards of proficiency for pre-registration midwifery education (NMC 2004a) and The Code. Standards of conduct, performance and ethics for nurses and midwives (NMC 2008). Consider which standards relate to the collection of specimens including vaginal swabs.

It is the responsibility of the midwife to identify any deviation from normal during pregnancy and refer immediately to an appropriate health professional (NMC 2004b:16). Therefore, it is the role of the midwife to collect specimens for diagnostic tests and to ensure that the appropriate procedure is followed. It is also important to prevent cross infection by adhering to universal precautions, to record tests taken and results obtained, and to ensure woman-centred care by involving clients in all aspects of their care journey.

In addition to the procedures described in Box 7.1, there are specific procedures for the collection of different specimens (see Box 7.2).

Box 7.1 Procedure for specimen collection

- **Check the client's case notes and medical record, in consultation with the client**
  Rationale To ascertain the type of specimen to be collected and why it is required. The client should be aware of the plan to undertake the test and what the result might mean
- **Explain the nature of the specimen and the procedure for its collection, and gain verbal consent from the client**
  Rationale The client should give clear consent to any procedure which involves you touching the client or obtaining a specimen from them. The client may take the specimen themselves and give it to you, which suggests they consent to the test. However, they should also understand what will happen to the specimen, how long the results are likely to take, and how they will find out about the results
- **Prepare equipment necessary to carry out the specimen collection: check the right container or medium for each specimen**
  Rationale To ensure ease of carrying out the procedure, and that the appropriate specimen is collected from the right part of the body utilizing the right container or transport medium
- **Label the containers/swabs with the patient information according to hospital policy**

Rationale To ensure the right tests are carried out for the right patient, and to minimize the potential distress of having to repeat the specimen collection
- **Wash hands**
  Rationale To avoid contamination of specimen container; to carry out clean procedure
- **Apply non-sterile gloves**
  Rationale To protect practitioner from infection risk presented by body fluids
- **Collect specimen (see procedure for individual specimen collection below)**
  Rationale To ensure adequate specimen sent for analysis
- **Remove gloves and wash hands**
  Rationale To reduce the risk of cross infection and/or contamination
- **Send specimen in appropriate, labelled envelope to correct department**
  Rationale To ensure speedy delivery of the specimen to the laboratory. To ensure correct analysis is carried out for the individual patient
- **Document the procedure in the maternity notes/medical notes and plan of care**
  Rationale To ensure good information sharing with other professionals; to keep a clear record of all care; to highlight in the plan of care the need to follow up results.

Box 7.2 Procedure for collection of high vaginal swabs

- **Explain how the procedure is carried out and reassure the client that privacy and dignity will be maintained**
  Rationale The client should feel safe and supported during the procedure and should be aware of measures taken to maintain privacy and dignity
- **Encourage the client to empty her bladder**
  Rationale To promote comfort during the procedure
- **Prepare equipment necessary: apron, sterile gloves; sterile VE pack; warm water; lubricating jelly; Cusco's speculum; absorbent disposable draw sheet; sterile vaginal swabs with transport medium**
  Rationale To ensure ease of carrying out the procedure, prevent cross-contamination of the swab; promote comfort of the woman
- **Position the woman in a recumbent position, on the absorbent sheet, ankles together and drawn up towards the body, knees open. Keep the lower body covered with a sheet until just before the swab is collected. Underwear should be removed**
  Rationale To ensure the swab is collected appropriately, and to maintain the woman's dignity and comfort during the procedure

- **Wash hands, open pack and drop sterile gloves onto the field. Wash hands again**
  Rationale To avoid contamination of specimen container; to carry out clean procedure
- **Apply sterile gloves**
  Rationale To protect the midwife from infection risk presented by body fluids; to prevent cross infection
- **Wash the vulva with swabs dipped in warm water, in a top to bottom direction.**
  Rationale To prevent cross-contamination
- **Lubricate speculum; part labia with non-dominant hand; insert speculum gently into the vagina sideways; rotate speculum 90 degrees and open; insert swab through speculum to top of vagina and rotate**
  Rationale To ensure adequate specimen sent for analysis
- **Remove gloves and wash hands**
  Rationale To reduce the risk of cross infection and/or contamination
- **Document the procedure in the maternity notes/medical notes and plan of care**
  Rationale To ensure good information sharing with other professionals; to keep a clear record of all care; to highlight in the plan of care the need to follow up results.

1. The midwife discusses the procedure with the woman enabling her to understand its relevance to her care and give consent

As with any procedure, no matter how familiar to the practitioner, the collection of specimens, particularly vaginal swabs, may be distressing to the client. Testing for certain conditions can cause anxiety on the part of the woman, for her own or her baby's health. The midwife can determine how well the client understands the procedure, and the reasons for it, through discussion, and through providing ample time for the woman to ask questions. The implications of abnormal values may require further explanation, such as in the case of GBS, where the woman may want to know what the risks to her baby are, and what treatment will be necessary if the results are positive.

2. The observation is made at the appropriate time according to the woman's plan of care

Midwives take specimens in a range of circumstances. She may have identified a possible infection as part of her planned care for the woman, in which case she will follow local guidelines regarding which tests to take and whom to notify. In other cases the woman may have a range of risk factors which fulfil the criteria for screening tests to be undertaken. The midwife may also be required to obtain specimens as a result of a request from another health professional. Whatever the rationale for the test, it should be clearly documented in the woman's maternity record why the test was taken, when and by whom. If tests are carried out according to a protocol or care pathway, this should be referred to and should also be documented.

3. The observation is made using the correct technique

The procedure for taking specimens is detailed in Box 7.1. The correct swab and medium should be identified for the particular test in mind. The woman should be made aware, when testing for a range of organisms, why more than one sample may be required.

4. The woman is supported during the observation and her reaction observed

Women may be distressed or embarrassed by the collection of the specimen. Stool specimens may be unpleasant to collect and transport; the procedure involved in the collection of vaginal swabs can be challenging, uncomfortable and can make women feel humiliated or self-conscious. The professional approach and clinical expertise of the midwife, along with a sensitive and supportive manner, may minimize some of these effects.

5. The woman is made comfortable after the measurement

Particularly in the case of vaginal swabs, the woman's dignity must be maintained throughout the procedure, and time should be taken afterwards to allow the woman to get comfortable and, if necessary, re-dress.

6. The woman is informed of the result

The woman should be aware of how long the results will take to be reported, and how she will be informed of the results. The implications of results should also be explained so that the client knows what to expect and is fully involved in her care.

7. If the result is outside normal parameters it is reported to an appropriate member of the team

Midwives must be aware of what the normal ranges of values are for the various specimens and tests that are being carried out, and to whom any abnormal results should be reported.

8. An accurate and legible record is made of the observation

All results should be recorded in black ink in the appropriate sections of the maternity record. Any treatments which occur based on the results should be documented and incorporated into a plan of care. Consultations with other professionals and instructions from obstetricians or GPs should also be recorded.

Reflection on trigger scenario

Revisit the trigger scenario from the beginning of the chapter.

Sascha was 32 weeks pregnant with her second baby, and had had Group B Streptococcus infection in her first pregnancy. She came into the delivery suite for a high vaginal swab. 'Why do I have to have this swab taken again?' Sascha asks. 'I had antibiotics last time, and the baby was okay. I really don't like having this done.'

This scenario relates to a woman with a risk of GBS in pregnancy, which could affect her baby after birth. However, there are many reasons why a midwife might collect specimens of body fluids or wastes from women in their care. This chapter has covered a range of other specimens which might be collected for diagnostic tests, and how these are collected. A further exploration of specimen collection is made using the jigsaw model.

Effective communication

There is a need for midwives to use a range of communication skills in this scenario. Sascha is understandably anxious about the procedure, and taking time to discuss her feelings and answer her questions should provide the support and information she needs to help alleviate her concerns. Some

questions the midwife might ask her include: What kind of experience did she have in her last pregnancy when having a HVS done? What is her understanding of the test and its implications? Focusing on the reason for the procedure should support Sascha in giving proper informed consent. Verbal reassurance about measures taken to ensure privacy might also be useful.

Effective communication with other professionals, including verbal and written communication, are an important part of the midwife's role in this scenario.

Woman-centred care

Focusing on woman-centred care for Sascha would mean that the midwife must take into account Sascha's feelings and fears about having a HVS taken and what the results might mean for her and her baby. Is the test truly necessary? Why is the test being carried out? Is this for Sascha's benefit or simply because hospital protocol requires the test to be done? Carrying out the test at a time that suits Sascha might support a more woman-centred approach. You might also ask how best to promote Sascha's comfort during the procedure. For example, some midwives, when using a metal speculum, warm the speculum before use, by placing it for a few moments in warm water. What safety issues might be raised by doing this?

Using best evidence

Using best evidence in relation to specimen collection means understanding the evidence which indicates the need for investigative tests for some women in certain circumstances, and understanding how these tests will promote maternal and fetal wellbeing. Evidence from the RCOG (2003), for example, shows that women should not be routinely screened for GBS in pregnancy, and that only those with a risk factor for the infection should be offered a HVS and treatment if the result is positive.

Professional and legal issues

The professional framework within which midwives work requires them to be competent in performing clinical tasks. It also requires that midwives refer women to an appropriate practitioner when a deviation from the norm is noted. The midwife cannot carry out such an invasive procedure without Sascha's informed consent, and this consent must be documented clearly in Sascha's maternity record. Questions you might ask are: Is it really necessary for Sascha to have this test? What issues are raised by this scenario in relation to the midwife's role? What would the midwife do if Sascha refused to have the test?

Team working

While the midwife might have carried out the HVS according to a hospital protocol, guideline or care pathway, she will not be working in isolation. She will consult with and inform her obstetric colleagues about the test and ensure that the result is communicated to them. Any ongoing care will be planned in consultation with the obstetric team. The collection of specimens means working in liaison with other professionals in microbiology, histology and other laboratory departments. How will the midwife communicate with these professionals? What systems are in

place to ensure that results are acted on appropriately. What other support services are involved in the collection of specimens?

Clinical dexterity

The procedure for specimen collection is described in Box 7.1, however there may be minor differences in the equipment used depending on the clinical area or hospital in which the midwife practises. For example, some Trusts might use re-usable metal speculums, while others use disposable plastic speculums for the procedure. Student midwives often work in a range of settings throughout their educational programme, necessitating becoming familiar with a range of local protocols. The midwife will need to be familiar with the equipment used for this procedure in her place of work, and should be able to use the speculum safely, effectively and without hesitation. The skills involved in this procedure include communication and psychological care as well as the physical requirements of the task. You might ask the following questions: How might a midwife become more dexterous in the use of the speculum and in carrying out the whole procedure? How might she promote comfort?

Models of care

The model of care being used should be woman-centred, but as mentioned above, midwives might also be bound by a range of hospital policies, protocols, guidelines or care pathways. In this case, the specimen collection will be part of the midwife's holistic care of Sascha at this point in her pregnancy. The midwife must negotiate between the institutional model of care and the midwifery approach that places the woman at the centre of care. As such, the procedure should be seen in relation to Sascha's whole pregnancy, and so questions should be asked about what interventions, if any, would follow a positive result, who will follow up the results and who will coordinate her care. Are women with complicated pregnancies where you work able to have midwifery led care?

Safe environment

Maintaining a safe environment involves ensuring that the woman is kept comfortable and has her dignity maintained at all times. The midwife is protected by wearing a protective apron and gloves, and by washing hands before and after the procedure. Other issues include the potential for others to enter the room, the safe transport of specimens, and the correct use of appropriate equipment. The correct disposal of waste is also an important issue when carrying out procedures involving body fluids or tissues.

Promotes health

In terms of promoting health, the woman might be concerned that the HVS might harm her baby. Clear explanation of the procedure should prevent any anxiety about this. The aim of the procedure is to promote health through early diagnosis of potential complications, and therefore this is a good chance to discuss with her and perhaps her partner just how such tests can prevent her baby developing a neonatal infection. How can the midwife determine Sascha's understanding of the procedure and the need to have the test carried out? What other opportunities does this situation present for health promotion? How does this test relate to future potential pregnancies?

Further scenarios

The following scenarios enable you to consider how specific situations influence the care the midwife provides. Consider the following in relation to the jigsaw model.

Scenario 1

Emma has been re-admitted to the delivery suite six days after a caesarean section. She is experiencing considerable discomfort at the wound site and has been wearing a sanitary pad over the site to absorb fluid loss from the wound. She is a large woman with a BMI of 35. She also complains of feeling unwell and has a temperature of 38.1°C. On examination, the wound is red, inflamed and tender to the touch, leaking haemoserous fluid.

Practice point

Wound infection is a potential complication of any surgery. The diagnosis of infection can be made through observation of the wound, the combination of symptoms, and through sending a wound swab to the laboratory for culture and sensitivity.

- Why do we need to send the wound swab to the lab if we can already see from an examination that the wound is infected?
- What are the risk factors for developing a postoperative infection, and which of these factors apply to Emma?
- Why is the wound leaking fluid?
- What compounding factors may have affected wound healing?
- What might be her plan of care?

Scenario 2

Baby Jonas was born 15 minutes ago. His mother Yasmin had prolonged rupture of the fetal membranes, and a slight pyrexia in labour. The neonatal Senior House Officer has requested that the baby has swabs taken to screen for infection.

Practice point

Babies born to women with evidence of chorioamnionitis should be referred to a neonatologist (NICE 2007) who is likely to request screening of the baby for infection. The places that swabs are taken are sites which might be colonized by infectious bacteria. Such infections are dangerous for the baby's immature immune system.

- What places would you need to take swabs from for an infection screen?
- What questions might Yasmin ask about this procedure?
- What midwifery skills might you employ in this situation in relation to supporting Yasmin?

- How might this screening influence the postnatal care of Yasmin and Jonas?

Conclusion

Collection of specimens for laboratory analysis and investigation is a very important aspect of the midwife's role, providing vital information about clients' health and indications for treatment and ongoing care. Midwives will be involved in identifying when specimens are required, either based on their own clinical judgement, the directions of medical and obstetric colleagues, or in accordance with hospital policies or care pathways. Therefore, midwives must develop the skills to carry out the procedures correctly, with minimal distress to mother or baby, and must be able to accurately label and dispatch specimens. Following up on results is also part of this process, in liaison with colleagues, and as part of her role of keeping women informed and supporting them as partners in their own care.

Useful resources

HealthcareAtoZ
http://www.healthcarea2z.org

HPA Guidance
www.hpa-standardmethods.org.uk/

Group B Strep Support
http://www.gbss.org.uk/?gclid=CK_Yye6PwY8CFQRIMAodO3bhPg

National Library for Health
http://www.library.nhs.uk/Default.aspx

Royal College of Obstetricians and Gynaecologists (RCOG) Prevention of early onset neonatal GBS
http://www.rcog.org.uk/index.asp?PageID=520

Women's health specialist library
http://www.library.nhs.uk/womenshealth/

References

Gilchrist B 2000 Taking a wound swab. Nursing Times 96(4 supp): 2

HPA 2005 Standard operating procedure for the investigation of gastric aspirates and infection screen swabs from neonates http://www.hpa-standardmethods.org.uk/documents/bsop/pdf/bsop23.pdf

Johnson R, Taylor W 2006 Skills for midwifery practice, 2nd edn. Elsevier, Edinburgh

McKay-Moffat S, Lee P 2006 A pocket guide for student midwives. Wiley, Chichester

Mallik M, Hall C, Howard. D (eds) 2004 Nursing knowledge and practice. Foundations for decision making, 2nd edn. Ballière Tindall, Edinburgh

Medforth J, Battersby S, Evans M et al 2006 Oxford handbook of midwifery. Oxford University Press, Oxford

National Institute for Health and Clinical Excellence (NICE) 2003 Antenatal care: routine care for the healthy pregnant woman. Clinical guideline 6. RCOG Press, London

National Institute for Health and Clinical Excellence (NICE) 2006 Routine postnatal care of women and their babies. NICE, London

National Institute for Health and Clinical Excellence (NICE) 2007 Intrapartum care. Care of healthy women and their babies during childbirth. NICE clinical guideline 55. NICE, London

Nursing and Midwifery Council (NMC) 2004a Standards of proficiency for pre-registration midwifery education. NMC, London

Nursing and Midwifery Council (NMC) 2004b Midwives rules and standards. NMC, London

Nursing and Midwifery Council (NMC) 2008 The Code. Standards of conduct, performance and ethics for nurses and midwives. NMC, London

RCOG 2003 Guideline No 36: Prevention of early onset Group B Streptrococcal disease. http://www.rcog.org.uk/resources/Public/pdf/GroupB_strep_no36.pdf

Timby B 2005 Fundemental nursing skills and concepts. Lippincott, Williams and Wilkins, Philadelphia

Chapter 8

Urinalysis

Introduction

This chapter focuses on one of the key skills required to assess the physical wellbeing of the woman or her baby. Urinalysis is the physical and chemical examination of urine, which is used to screen for disease or infections or to manage an underlying condition. The midwife needs to know why and when this test is to be carried out, and what may affect changes in urine constitution in pregnancy and for the neonate. S/he also needs to be able to carry out urinalysis appropriately and understand the significance of the results.

Trigger scenario

Consider the following scenario in relation to urinalysis and what you need to know to help you interpret the situation.

Fatima is 30 weeks pregnant with her third baby, attending her local antenatal clinic. She says she is feeling faint at the moment and larger this time than she remembered with her previous children. Isobel the midwife tests Fatima's urine and discovers that there are ketones in it. She turns to Fatima and asks, 'What did you eat for breakfast?'

What do you need to know in order to interpret this situation? Reflecting on this scenario you may have asked yourself:

- What is the relevance of Fatima feeling larger this pregnancy?
- Why was the midwife testing her urine?
- How did she test Fatima's urine?
- What was she testing her urine for?
- What is the relevance of ketones in urine?
- What are the predisposing factors?
- What should the midwife do having discovered ketones in Fatima's urine?
- What is the relevance of asking Fatima what she had for breakfast?
- How does pregnancy affect the constituents of urine?

Background physiology

The formation of urine

The production of urine is the result of the body's need to maintain an appropriate environment for optimum function of the systems of the body. The body must excrete the waste products of metabolism whilst maintaining essential constituents and managing the balance of water. For example, the concentration of urine varies depending on the needs of the body. On a hot day, when a woman loses fluid through perspiration, and has had little to drink, the body still attempts to conserve fluid by producing dark, concentrated urine. The constituents of urine also reflect potential pathology. Urine does not normally contain glucose or protein, for example, however there are situations that make such an observation more likely.

Urine is formed as blood flows through the kidneys. The kidneys are composed of approximately one million nephrons, the functional units responsible for the filtration of blood. This production of urine is a complex process that can be divided into three steps:

1. Filtration

This occurs in the glomerulus (a coil of capillaries) from which water and other substances in the blood are forced out under pressure into the Bowman's capsule (a tube, the closed end of which surrounds the glomerulus, the open end leads to the urinary collecting ducts and the renal pelvis).

Activity

Access an anatomy text to find a picture of a Bowman's capsule or look at the diagram at http://en.wikipedia. org/wiki/Bowman's_capsule.

Substances with a molecular mass of greater than 68 kilodaltons (kDa) remain in the capillary (Coad 2006). The rate at which blood is filtered by both kidneys is the glomerular filtration rate (GFR) and this is about 120 ml per minute (Blows 2001).

2. Re-absorption

This selective reabsorption returns all the glucose and amino acids to the capillaries surrounding the nephron. The amount of water that returns to the blood is controlled by the antidiuretic hormone (ADH) and the reabsorption of sodium is controlled by aldosterone. Calcium and phosphate reabsorption is controlled by the hormone calcitonin.

3. Secretion

Potassium, ammonia and hydrogen ions are actively secreted into the renal tubule from the capillaries. Drugs and toxins may also enter the filtrate by this process (Coad 2006). The end product is now urine, which collects in the renal pelvis and is conducted via the ureters to the bladder. Urine is voided from the bladder via the urethra.

Physiology in relation to pregnancy

There are a number of changes that take place in the urinary system during pregnancy that may have an impact on the production and constitution of urine.

- The kidneys enlarge in weight and size with dilatation of the renal pelves and calyces.
- The ureters dilate and stretch, leading to curving.
- Relaxation of the muscles of the internal urethral sphincter takes place.
- The glomerular filtration rate increases leading to greater amounts of urea, creatinine, glucose and folate being excreted.
- Reduction of bladder capacity.
- Urine may be more alkaline.

Activity

Access an anatomy textbook and consider which hormones or other factors may cause the above.

The composition of urine

Urine is 96% water, 4% dissolved substances (Johnson & Taylor 2006). Urinalysis is performed to detect the presence, or measure the value, of the potential constituents of the sample.

Specific gravity

The ability of the kidneys to concentrate urine is reflected by this test. It measures how much more dense the urine is compared to water (Blows 2001). The normal range for specific gravity is 1.002–1.030 (McKinney et al 2000); the higher the value, the more concentrated the urine.

Acidity – pH

Urine is less acidic (higher pH) when a urinary tract infection is present. Acidic urine predisposes to the formation of kidney stones (Johnson & Taylor 2006). Normal pH is between 4.6 and 8.0 (McKinney et al 2000).

Protein

There should be no protein in urine. A positive result may indicate infection, contamination or developing pre-eclampsia. Further tests would be indicated to assess the amount of protein and the presence of infection. Early morning specimens are more concentrated and are most appropriate for the detection of protein. In pregnancy, due to the action of progesterone, the ureters become distended and tortuous. Compounded by compression from the enlarged ovarian arteries and veins and the gravid uterus, there is urinary stasis in the ureters, increasing the risk of infection (Coad 2006). Pre-eclampsia is a potentially life-threatening condition requiring close monitoring (Lewis 2007).

Blood

There should be no blood in urine. A positive result may indicate infection, trauma (following catheterization for example) or contamination and requires further investigation.

Glucose

There should be no glucose in urine. During pregnancy, however, there is a tendency for glomerular filtration to exceed the renal threshold for glucose and glycosuria results (Blows 2001). Assessment of glucose in urine is currently not recommended (NICE 2008). However, practitioners should be aware of those women who may be at risk of diabetes. Ideally all women should have had pre-conception assessment to establish if they are diabetic or have a family history of the condition. However, most women will not have had this opportunity and establishing appropriate screening for diabetes in pregnancy is currently being developed (NICE 2007a).

Activity

Find out what macrosomia means and what risks there are to the baby if a woman develops diabetes in pregnancy.

Ketones

There should be no ketones in urine. Ketones are formed following the breakdown of fat. They may be present if the woman has not been eating (during prolonged labour) or has been vomiting excessively (hyperemesis gravidarum). Women with uncontrolled diabetes may also have ketonuria. Links have been made between maternal ketonuria among women with post-term pregnancy and an increased rate of oligohydramnios and fetal heart rate anomalies (Onyeije & Dixon 2001).

Nitrites

There should he no nitrites in urine. They are produced by bacteria and are therefore suggestive of infection (McKinney et al 2000).

Bilirubin

There should be no bilirubin in urine. Its presence may indicate hepatic disease and requires further investigation. A false negative result may occur if the sample is exposed to sunlight (Johnson & Taylor 2006).

Urobilinogen

This is normally present in urine in small amounts, 0.09–4.23 μmol in 24 hours (Blows 2001) but raised levels are suggestive of excessive haemolysis or liver disease.

Activity

What is the place of laboratory urine testing in the treatment of substance abuse?

National guidance

The current NICE Guidelines for antenatal care indicate that urinalysis for proteinuria should be carried out at each antenatal appointment (NICE 2008). Further screening for asymptomatic bacteriuria, a factor involved in preterm birth, should be offered at an early stage in pregnancy (Smaill 2007, NICE 2008).

Activity

Access the Action on Pre-eclampsia PECOG guidelines at http://www.apec.org.uk/guidelines.htm and consider those on urinalysis. Are these guidelines followed in your area of work?

It is not recommended to screen for diabetes routinely, by testing for glucose in the urine, though this is sometimes the practice (Anderson 2007). Within the guidelines for intrapartum care, urinalysis is included as part of the initial assessment of labour, with regularly ensuring the woman empties her bladder throughout the first stage (NICE 2007b). There is no specific guidance relating to urinalysis in the NICE guidelines for postnatal care (NICE 2006), although a midwife should use professional judgement if either a woman or a baby are suspected to be unwell and a urinary tract infection (UTI) is suspected.

Professional guidelines

Midwives must work within the professional framework of the Nursing and Midwifery Council in order to practise in the United Kingdom.

Activity

Access the Standards of proficiency for pre-registration midwifery education (NMC 2004a) and The Code. Standards of conduct, performance and ethics for nurses and midwives (NMC 2008) performance and ethics. Consider which standards are relevant to the issue of testing urine.

The Midwives rules and standards (NMC 2004b) outline the responsibility of midwives to recognize any deviation from normal in either the woman or the baby and to refer such cases to an appropriate health professional. The midwife is also responsible for monitoring antenatal, intrapartum and postnatal progress and this includes undertaking urinalysis in line with local and national guidelines.

Urinalysis

Urinalysis generally refers to the activity involving the immersion of a reagent strip into a specimen of urine followed by visual interpretation of the results. The accuracy of this method has come into question and automated analysis may be more appropriate in some situations (Waugh et al 2005). However, urine is also examined through observation and the use of smell, and under the microscope in a laboratory. The reagent strips may be for the detection of a single substance, such as glucose, or have multiple test pads on a single strip. There is a range

of products on the market and each surgery or Hospital Trust will purchase reagents that meet the needs of their clients and budgets.

Activity

Find out which types of reagent strips are available in your clinical area and find out what they test for and why.

Urinalysis is performed on a range of samples:

Early morning specimen of urine (EMU)

Urine is collected during the first visit of the day to the toilet. This specimen is the most concentrated of the day, thus enhancing the detection of solutes such as protein and hormones.

Midstream specimen of urine (MSU)

The woman is asked to start urinating in the toilet and then to catch some urine in a clean container (sterile if going to the laboratory). The bladder is then completely emptied in the toilet. This specimen should therefore be free from contamination from the urethra as the urine that first flushes through is not collected for examination.

Catheter specimen of urine (CSU)

Women may have a urinary catheter in situ following surgery or epidural analgesia. Bacteria may have been introduced into the urinary tract increasing the risk of infection and a sample of urine may be required for analysis in the laboratory. If the urinary catheter is draining freely a small clamp is applied to the proximal end of the drainage tube (not the catheter) for 30 minutes to allow urine to build up in the tube. Some catheter drainage bags have a latex port which require a needle and syringe to aspirate a urine sample. Another type of bag has a port onto which a syringe can be attached directly. Ensuring that the woman's privacy is maintained, the port should be swabbed with an alcohol wipe and allowed to dry. Wearing gloves, the practitioner aspirates urine from the port and transfers the specimen to a sterile specimen bottle. The clamp is then removed.

Activity

Locate the types of catheters and drainage systems available in your place of work. Consider how you would obtain a specimen.

Find out in what circumstances catheter specimens are obtained.

24-hour urine collection

The collection begins at a suitable time during the day, such as 10.00 hours, and at this time, the woman is asked to empty her bladder in the toilet. Every subsequent time that she voids urine in the next 24 hours, she collects it in a jug and then pours it into a large screwtop container. At the time at which the collection began 24 hours previously the woman collects her final urine sample and this is then added to the collection.

Activity

Find out what the following terms mean:
Dysuria, frequency of micturition, polyuria, glycosuria, urgency of micturition.

Observation of urine

Urine is usually clear, although it may become cloudy if left to stand. Urine may also appear cloudy if there is a urinary tract infection. Normally, urine is described as being straw coloured (Johnson & Taylor 2006) but the strength of colour will vary depending on the concentration. It may be coloured pink if there is blood present. It should also he noted that the consumption of beetroot may also have a similar effect. The urine of the neonate may leave a pink stain on the nappy. This is caused by the deposit of urate crystals and is normal (Gorrie, McKinney & Murray 1998). Dark concentrated urine is an indication of dehydration, whereas a yellow/orange colour may indicate the presence of bilirubin. Urine does not normally have a strong smell but if there is infection present it may have a distinctive fishy odour. The presence of ketones in urine may lead to a smell similar to that of pear drops. Some foods, such as asparagus, also leave their smell in urine.

Equipment for urinalysis

Historically midwives may have learnt how to carry out urinalysis using chemical reagents. However, in the majority of cases it is now possible to test using reagent sticks. There are many types of these available and you should be aware of those used in your locality.

Activity

Identify which reagent sticks are used in your area. Read the instructions to establish:

- what these test for
- how long you need to place these in the urine
- how long you should wait prior to reading the results.

In situations where more accuracy is required, such as in hypertension, more specific laboratory or electronic testing may be required (Waugh et al 2005).

1. The midwife discusses the procedure with the woman enabling her to understand its relevance to her care and give consent

Any procedure, no matter how familiar to the practitioner, may cause anxiety in clients. Many women may never have had a urine test prior to pregnancy and will need reassurance and explanation of the need for the test (see Box 8.1). The practitioner can ascertain if the woman is familiar with the procedure through simple questioning, avoiding inappropriately lengthy explanations. It may be helpful to show her what the reagent sticks look like.

Box 8.1 Procedure of urinalysis

- **Consult the client's plan of care**
  Rationale To ensure that the client's condition is monitored effectively. The client should be sufficiently involved in her care that she is expecting to have her urine tested
- **Gain verbal consent from the client**
  Rationale To ensure that the client's condition is monitored effectively. The client should be sufficiently involved in her care that she is expecting to have her urine tested
- **Gain verbal consent from the client**
  Rationale The fact that the woman has produced a specimen of urine and given it to you, implies that she consents to having it tested. However, it is essential that the women knows what it is being tested for, not least to avoid embarrassment when results are given, but more importantly, to avoid

the possibility of a breakdown in trust that may occur when information is withheld
- **Assess the possibility of confounding factors**
  Rationale To avoid the possibility of contamination, and to ensure results reflect the true clinical picture
- **Locate appropriate urine sticks**
  Rationale To undertake required urinalysis, avoiding omission or duplication
- **Check expiry date of urine sticks**
  Rationale To achieve accurate results
- **Wash hands**
  Rationale To avoid contamination of urine stick
- **Apply non-sterile gloves**
  Rationale To protect practitioner from infection risk presented by body fluids

continued

Box 8.1 continued

- **Immerse urine stick in specimen, remove and leave for required length of time, according to test and manufacturer's instruction**
  Rationale To apply urine evenly to reagent on urine strip. Each individual test on the urine stick will take a varying length of time to complete. The practitioner must make herself familiar with each test and the product supplied for use in her area of practice
- **Dispose of stick and urine in line with local policy**
  Rationale Each Trust will have a policy for the disposal of clinical waste. Urine must never be poured down the sink: a

designated sluice should be used where available. In an outpatient setting, clients may wish to wash and re-use the bottle, and it may be secured and returned for this purpose
- **Remove gloves and wash hands**
  Rationale To reduce the risk of cross infection and/or contamination
- **Inform the client of the result of the urinalysis**
  Rationale To involve the client in her care
- *Document the results*
  Rationale To ensure continuity, completeness and compliance with professional standards.

Questioning is likely to focus on whether the urine test is normal. Midwives should therefore be familiar with normal testing values for women and babies. The implications of abnormal values need careful explanation.

2. The observation is made at the appropriate time according to the woman's plan of care

Where urinalysis forms part of an individual plan of care this should he clearly documented and evaluated. Women should be assessed individually for their needs but the general guidance is in Box 8.2.

3. The observation is made using the correct technique

Women should he informed that urine specimens for urinalysis in the antenatal period should ideally be collected at the first visit to the toilet that

day; and that specimens should be collected midstream to avoid contamination. The midwife should be aware of the different reagent sticks available and check the appropriate method of use before testing. Box 8.1 explains how to carry out the testing.

4. The woman is supported during the observation and her reaction observed

Women do not generally have problems collecting urine samples. However, it may be a source of embarrassment for some, and practitioners need to be discrete. During a 24-hour urine collection, provision should he made for safe and hygienic storage.

Activity

Find out what 24-hour urine specimens are tested for. Why are they collected? What is an abnormal result?

Box 8.2 Rationale for undertaking urinalysis at different stages

Antenatal period Urinalysis is part of routine antenatal care. Women will be asked for a midstream specimen of urine at the booking visit and at each subsequent antenatal examination. This enables a baseline to be established and detection of other conditions requiring further investigation. Any antenatal admission to hospital or physical cause for concern, including abdominal pain, labour, rupture of membranes, antepartum haemorrhage, etc. would necessitate repeating urinalysis to exclude underlying pathology.

Intrapartum period At the onset of labour urinalysis is undertaken in order to detect any condition that may impact on the progress of labour. When labour is prolonged, urinalysis should continue in order to detect any developing abnormality. Ketosis may be a sign of dehydration and proteinurea may be indicative of the development of pre-eclampsia or infection.

Postnatal period Urinalysis is not normally indicated in the postnatal period when women have had a normal birth and there are no other complications suggestive of urinary tract involvement. It is policy in many Hospital Trusts that a specimen of urine should be taken prior to the removal of a urinary catheter. This specimen would be examined in the laboratory, to identify underlying infection.

The midwife will undertake urinalysis if there is any unexplained deterioration in a woman's condition postnatally or where infection is suspected, for example pyrexia, dysuria, or abdominal tenderness.

Neonatal period Urinalysis is rarely undertaken on neonates in the postnatal period. It may be indicated as part of an infection screen for congenital abnormality of the urinary tract. Collecting a urine specimen from an infant requires the application of a specially designed, single use collection bag. Care is taken to involve parents in the procedure as it takes careful monitoring of the baby to achieve the necessary sample. The skin should be clean and dry and the bag attached to the perineum, avoiding leaving any gaps through which urine could escape. The nappy can be reapplied following the addition of a slit through which the bag can be passed, enabling the sample to be seen as soon as possible.

5. The woman is made comfortable after the measurement

The comfort of the woman should not be compromised during this procedure.

6. The woman is informed of the result

If the result is in the normal range this should be indicated to the woman. If results are outside the normal range the significance of this should be explained

to her carefully, especially in relation to her baby, as it may cause her anxiety.

7. If the result is outside normal parameters it is reported to an appropriate member of the team

As indicated above midwives should understand the significance of urinalysis ranges in pregnant and postnatal women. If the values fall outside what is regarded as normal she should inform a registered practitioner and other relevant members of the midwifery team of her findings.

8. An accurate and legible record is made of the observation

Readings must be recorded on the appropriate documentation, in black ink. Where any action was taken as a result of the urinalysis, this should also be documented and a plan of care developed.

Activity

What does NAD mean?

Reflection on trigger scenario

Reconsider the trigger scenario at the start

Fatima is 30 weeks pregnant with her third baby, attending her local antenatal clinic. She says she is feeling faint at the moment and larger this time than she remembered with her previous children. Isobel the midwife tests Fatima's urine and discovers that there are ketones in it. She turns to Fatima and asks, 'What did you eat for breakfast?'

The scenario relates to a woman during pregnancy. It is more likely that the midwife will need to test urine more frequently during the antenatal period. This chapter has explored some of the physiological and psychological issues around caring for women in this situation and you will have more insight into the issues in the scenario. The jigsaw model will be used to consider the issues in more depth.

Effective communication

Midwives consistently need to use appropriate communication skills in maternity care to ensure the psychological wellbeing of the woman. In an antenatal clinic, where midwives may have only short periods of allocated time, effective and skilled communication is very important. The midwife will need to be especially aware of appropriate questioning techniques and listening skills. Further, how Isobel records the information is important. Some questions that could arise include: Is this the first time Isobel and Fatima have met in this pregnancy? What information should Isobel give about urinalysis and its meaning? How and why did Isobel ask the question about breakfast? Is Fatima showing signs of fainting and how will Isobel respond to this? What information will be gained by Fatima recalling her breakfast? How will Isobel record the result obtained?

Woman-centred care

A woman-centred approach to this procedure would have been to look at the whole pattern of care required by Isobel to meet Fatima's needs. Asking what Fatima has had for breakfast shows Isobel has considered the wider perspective of why ketones have appeared in the urine. Questions that may arise include: Is Fatima's usual diet significant in the presence of ketones? Are there social issues affecting her dietary intake? Are there any other reasons why she may not be eating? Are there any medical causes for her having ketones? What effect does this have on her baby? What other observations may need to be carried out?

Using best evidence

In this situation providing effective care will be based on which method of urine testing is the most appropriate to use. However, the midwife may be reliant on particular urine test equipment provided by her Trust. Some questions that could arise are: Is the urine test reliable? Should she send the sample for further testing? When should she test Fatima's urine again?

Professional and legal issues

Midwives must practise within a professional and legal framework. Questions that may arise from this scenario are: Is Isobel following current guidelines in her assessment of Fatima's urine? Are there any external Trust issues that are affecting her timing of testing the urine? Is she using the correct equipment in the correct way? Are the guidelines in the hospital the same as those in primary care? What opportunities are there to keep up to date with new techniques and reagents?

Team working

Though a midwife tends to work on her own in a community clinic there will be others in her team area that will need to know information about abnormal results. Questions that may arise include: Where will the results of this be recorded? When should the urine test be repeated if at all? Who will need to be informed about this and how? What is the procedure for referral to a medical practitioner if necessary?

Clinical dexterity

The process of testing urine is described above; however the equipment required will depend on the individual Trust and clinical situation. The midwife will need to be familiar with all equipment devices used for urinalysis in her locality. The skills required for testing urine involve communication and

psychological care as well as the physical requirements of the task. Questions that may arise include: Is Isobel familiar with the equipment available. If she is not how should she find out how to use it? Are the test reagents out of date?

Models of care

Individual Trusts may organize antenatal services differently. In this scenario Isobel may be caring for Fatima as part of her case load as a midwife or for a colleague as part of a team. In a holistic woman-centred approach as indicated above, urinalysis will be completed as part of a whole person approach, considering all the aspects of Fatima's condition at the time. Questions that may arise include: If whole person care is being carried out how should Isobel approach the issue of testing Fatima's urine? How will the results affect the type of care given to an individual woman?

Safe environment

Antenatal care takes place in a range of environments, as part of a hospital base or a primary care unit, or in a woman's home. Consideration should be taken to the potential contamination of body fluids, including urine. Questions that could be asked include: How may the urine test be carried out with minimal risk of contamination to the midwife or the woman? Could the woman test it herself? Are there appropriate facilities for disposal? Are there appropriate facilities for handwashing? What are the procedures in case of spillage?

Promotes health

Midwives have an opportunity with each encounter to promote health and wellbeing for the woman and her baby. In this situation Isobel could use the opportunity to find out more about Fatima's lifestyle and social world in order to carry out appropriate assessment of her whole wellbeing. Questions that arise are: How may Isobel use this opportunity to promote health and wellbeing regarding the results found in her urine? What dietary advice can be offered in pregnancy?

Further scenarios

The following scenarios enable you to consider how specific situations influence the care the midwife provides. Use the jigsaw model to explore the issues raised in each scenario.

Scenario 1

At an antenatal appointment Tina, who is 35 weeks pregnant with her first baby, provides a sample of urine for testing. Clare, her midwife, observes that it looks a bit cloudy, and on removal of the lid, notices it has a strong odour. She asks Tina if she has been feeling well and Tina replies that, apart from some backache, she has been fine.

Practice point

In the antenatal period some women may be susceptible to urinary tract infections. Definitive diagnosis is usually through sending a midstream specimen to the laboratory for microscopic examination. However, there may be alternative reasons for urine to be visually contaminated or for other symptoms.

- What questions may Clare ask Tina about the urine container and why?
- Why does she ask Tina if she has been feeling well?

- What are the alternative diagnoses for cloudy urine?
- What other observations may she make on Tina to aid in her diagnosis?
- What may she expect to find on urinalysis and why?
- If she finds any changes on urine testing what will she do now?
- Where will she document her findings?

Scenario 2

Simone has had an emergency caesarean section two hours before. She has an intravenous infusion in her arm and a urinary catheter is in place, draining into a bag. Mandy, the midwife, observes there is a minimal amount in the bag and it looks very dark in colour.

Practice point

The pelvic anatomies are close together and in emergency situations, where a baby may need to be born quickly, the urinary tract may occasionally be damaged. Physiologically there is an expectation that women will have a diuresis in the initial period following birth. If this does not happen there may be a number of reasons and the midwife should be aware of what these reasons may be.

- What could be the possible causes of there being only a small amount of urine in the catheter bag?
- What are the reasons for the urine being dark in colour?
- What other observations may Mandy carry out to assess Simone's wellbeing?
- Where will she record her observations?
- Whom will she advise of her observations?
- What actions may need to be taken?

Conclusion

Urinalysis is an important aspect of the midwife's role, providing her with information regarding the woman's current health status. The midwife must identify when urinalysis is indicated, develop the skill of performing it accurately and consider how abnormal results are managed. The woman must remain central to this important screening test, with information not only provided but also interpreted.

Useful resources

Action on pre-eclampsia
http://www.apec.org.uk/pdf/
guidelinepublishedvers04.pdf

National Library for Health
http://www.library.nhs.uk/Default.aspx

Women's health specialist library
http://www.library.nhs.uk/
womenshealth/

References

Anderson T 2007 Sugar and spice and all things NICE. The Practising Midwife 10(3): 50

Blows W T 2001 The biological basis of nursing: clinical observations. Routledge, London

Coad J 2006 Anatomy and physiology for midwives, 2nd edn. Mosby, Edinburgh

Confidential Enquiry into Maternal and Child Health 2007 Perinatal mortality 2005: England, Wales and Northern Ireland. CEMACH, London

Gorrie T M, McKinney E S, Murray S S 1998 Clinical manual for foundations of maternal-newborn nursing, 2nd edn. WB Saunders, Philadelphia

Johnson R, Taylor W 2006 Skills for midwifery practice, 2nd edn. Churchill Livingstone, Edinburgh

Lewis G (ed) 2007 Confidential enquiry into maternal and child health. Why mothers die 2000–2002: The Sixth Report of the Confidential Enquiries into Maternal Deaths in the United Kingdom. CEMACH, London

McKinney E S, Ashwill J W, Murray S S et al 2000 Maternal-child nursing. WE Saunders, Philadelphia

National Institute for Health and Clinical Excellence (NICE) 2006 Routine postnatal care of women and their babies. NICE, London

National Institute for Health and Clinical Excellence (NICE) 2007a Diabetes in pregnancy: management of diabetes and its complications from pre-conception to the postnatal period. Online. Available: http://guidance.nice.org.uk/page.aspx?o=451295 13 Sep 2007

National Institute for Health and Clinical Excellence (NICE) 2007b Intrapartum care of healthy women and their babies during childbirth. NICE, London

National Institute for Health and Clinical Excellence (NICE) 2008 Antenatal care: Routine care for the healthy pregnant woman: clinical guideline 62. RCOG Press, London

Nursing and Midwifery Council (NMC) 2004a Standards of proficiency for pre-registration midwifery education. NMC, London

Nursing and Midwifery Council (NMC) 2004b Midwives rules and standards. NMC, London

Nursing and Midwifery Council (NMC) 2008 The Code. Standards of conduct, performance and ethics for nurses and midwives. NMC, London

Onyeije C I, Divon M Y 2001 The impact of maternal ketonuria on fetal test results in the setting of post term pregnancy. American Journal of Obstetrics and Gynecology 184(4): 713–718

Smaill F 2007 Asymptomatic bacteriuria in pregnancy. Best Practice and Research Clinical Obstetrics & Gynaecology 21(3): 439–450

Waugh J S, Bell S C, Kilby M D et al 2005 Optimal bedside urinalysis for the detection of proteinuria in hypertensive pregnancy: a study of diagnostic accuracy. BJOG: An International Journal of Obstetrics and Gynaecology 112(4): 412–417

Chapter 9

Venepuncture

Introduction

Venepuncture is the practice of taking blood from a vein. There are a number of reasons why a woman might need to have blood taken, and a range of tests that are common practice during pregnancy. Midwives need the practical skills to carry out the procedure, and an understanding of the range of tests and the reasons why these are performed for pregnant women.

Trigger scenario

Consider the following scenario in relation to venepuncture and what you need to know to help you interpret the situation.

Emily blinked to find the student peering over her. It was impossible to tell who was the most pale. 'You fainted', the student explained, looking as though she might do the same. 'Oh, I always do that when I have blood taken', Emily whispered, taking a sip from the water that had been thrust into her hand. 'I should have warned you.'

Questions from trigger

- Why might the student midwife be taking blood?
- Why might Emily have fainted?
- Could the student midwife have prevented Emily from fainting?
- What action could the student take to minimize the risk of Emily fainting again during venepuncture?

Background physiology

Before a student attempts to take blood, it is important that she has a basic understanding of the system that transports blood around the body.

Blood vessels

There are three types of blood vessels:

Arteries are large vessels that carry oxygenated blood away from the heart to the tissues. Arterioles are small arteries that deliver blood to the capillaries.

Capillaries are microscopic vessels that connect arterioles and venules.

They are so narrow that a red blood cell may have to fold to pass through them (Rankin 2005). They are found close to almost every cell in the body, permitting the exchange of gases, nutrients and waste. Venules (where several capillaries unite) collect blood from capillaries and drain it into veins.

Veins return blood to the heart from the capillary network. They have a thinner vessel wall than arteries and are the vessels from which blood is taken for laboratory analysis.

> **Activity**
>
> Find out which three layers of tissue make up the vessel walls of arteries and veins. How does the distribution of these three layers differ between arteries and veins?

The veins of the arm are divided into two groups: deep and superficial. The superficial veins which run along the antecubital fossa (inside the elbow) provide the best location for venepuncture.

Changes in pregnancy

During pregnancy there is an increase in blood volume and cardiac output accommodated by a decrease in peripheral resistance (Stables & Rankin 2005). Progesterone relaxes the smooth muscle that surrounds the walls of the veins, leading to vasodilation. Thus pregnant women often have excellent veins for venepuncture purposes.

Venepuncture

Venepuncture generally refers to the activity involving the puncture of a vein with a needle to take a sample of blood for analysis in the laboratory. You may come across the term phlebotomy: phleb = vein and otomy = cut into. It is a procedure that may be undertaken at any point in the childbirth continuum, depending on the condition of the woman; however, there are particular points throughout pregnancy when blood analysis is indicated.

> **Activity**
>
> Find out which blood tests are taken routinely during pregnancy. What are the normal values for these tests? What antenatal screening tests are offered to all women in your locality?

Equipment

There are two main ways in which blood is taken: using a needle and a syringe or using a vacuum system.

Needle and syringe

This system involves the use of a sterile needle and syringe to extract blood from the vein. Sterile, disposable needles are used and the practitioner should check that the seal on the package is unbroken. The size of the syringe should correspond to the amount of blood required and a 21 gauge (green) needle should be used (Johnson & Taylor 2006). The needle should be attached to the syringe, cover intact, before attending to the client to avoid causing unnecessary anxiety. The plunger of the syringe should be withdrawn very slightly as this will enable 'flash back' (when blood is seen at the tip of the syringe, confirming that a vein has been punctured) to be observed.

When a number of tests are required, it is necessary to transfer blood from the syringe to the individual specimen bottles. This method is potentially hazardous to the practitioner, who may sustain a needle stick injury during the process.

Vacuum system

This system includes a needle that attaches to a disposable plastic cuff into which a pre-vacuumed bottle is connected. When more than one blood sample is required, the needle remains in the vein and bottles are interchanged into the cuff. Blood does not seep out of the cuff during this process as there is a rubber sheath covering the cuff end of the needle that retracts back over the needle when the bottle is removed. The vacuum system has specifically designed needles that have two covered ends. The shortest (white) end is removed first and attached to the plastic cuff, using a screw action. The cover to the sharp end of the needle (green) remains intact until just before venepuncture takes place to keep the needle free from contamination.

Blood bottles

Each individual blood test requires a specific amount of whole blood or serum. Therefore a specific specimen bottle is required for each test. The bottles are colour coded and may contain a medium that enables the blood to be transported to the laboratory in optimum condition for subsequent analysis; for example, to prevent it from clotting. The pre-vacuumed bottles are also primed to take the required amount of blood, and therefore stop filling when an adequate sample has been withdrawn. So, for example, the bottle used to take blood for random blood sugar analysis (RBS) is small and stops filling very quickly, whereas the bottle used for a full blood count (FBC) is larger and fills almost to the top. Blood bottles have an expiry date and this should be checked prior to use.

Activity

Find out what colour bottles are required for each of the routine blood tests taken throughout the childbirth continuum.

Alcohol swab

The skin should be thoroughly cleaned prior to puncture and it is recommended that this should be with a 70% alcohol solution and allowed to dry for 30 seconds (Beyea & Nicoll 1996). To prevent re-contamination, the vein should not be palpated after swabbing.

Tourniquet

A tourniquet is an elasticated band used to achieve venous pooling, making the vein distended and more readily targeted. It is applied to the upper arm about 10 cm from the antecubital fossa (inside of the elbow). It should not be so tight that it stops arterial blood flow, causing the arm to change colour. The veins can be made more prominent by asking the woman to clench and unclench her fist, as the muscle action will encourage venous return. It is worth spending time locating the most suitable vein rather than literally 'having a stab at it'. The best vein is not always the largest or most visible. Students can develop the skill of palpating a vein using the pad of the index finger, feeling the springy nature of the vein beneath the skin. The student is advised to become familiar with the various types of tourniquet, ensuring that s/he knows how to release it using one hand. Many commercial companies provide tourniquets to professionals as a means of advertising their products. Ensure that you are not breaking local policy by inadvertently promoting baby milk companies, for example.

Non-sterile gloves

Local policy will probably require you to wear gloves for this procedure to prevent cross infection from client to the practitioner. All body fluids should be regarded as a source of potential infection and direct contact with them should be prevented where possible. Wearing gloves will not prevent needle stick injury, however, and measures should be taken to minimize this risk.

Activity

Find out what the local policy is regarding the action to be taken following needle stick injury.

Sharps box

A sharps box is a specially designed repository for contaminated needles and broken glass ampoules. They come in a range of sizes and are located in clinical rooms in hospital and community clinics, in a place that is out of reach to members of the public and especially of small children. You should take a sharps box with you to undertake venepuncture, to avoid the hazard of transporting used needles. The needle should not be removed from the syringe but placed in the sharps box as a unit.

It is important that the box does not become over-full as there may be a temptation to apply pressure in order to fit the syringe in the box, potentially resulting in injury from the contents. Never re-sheath a needle as this may result in a needle stick injury.

Additional equipment

You will also need: cotton wool ball (to apply to the puncture site to aid haemostasis), an adhesive dressing (to cover puncture site) and a clean metal or plastic receiver (cardboard trays are not appropriate as they are often re-used but not washable and therefore become a potential source of cross infection).

Procedure

This clinical skill requires considerable dexterity and confidence. It is advisable that the student does not attempt this procedure until she has observed the technique many times. S/he can begin to gain competence by identifying and gathering the necessary equipment and filling out the appropriate laboratory blood forms. S/he can practise identifying suitable veins by applying a tourniquet to fellow students or obliging midwives. Ideally s/he should have the opportunity to practise handling the equipment in a clinical simulation unit, before attempting the procedure on a woman. S/he must work under the direct supervision of a registered midwife until competent and confident. The student must be mindful not to undertake any duty that she is not trained to perform (NMC 2004).

The procedure for taking venous blood from an adult is described using the framework outlined in the introductory chapter. See Box 9.1 for an outline of the procedure for venepuncture.

Box 9.1 Procedure for venepuncture

■ **Consult the client's plan of care**
Rationale To ensure that the client's condition is monitored effectively

■ **Gain verbal consent from the client**
Rationale To ensure that the woman understands what the test involves and what the implications of the result might be

■ **Discuss the procedure with the client, identify the best arm to use**
Rationale To allay fears and correct misconceptions. To identify problems the client may have had with the procedure in the past, involving the client in her care

■ **Assess the possibility of confounding factors**
Rationale To avoid the possibility of contamination and ensure that the results reflect the true clinical picture

■ **Identify the appropriate blood bottles and gather equipment**
Rationale To ensure the correct bottles for specific test(s) are used. To have all equipment to hand thus avoiding having to leave the client or prolong the procedure

■ **Check expiry date of bottles**
Rationale To achieve accurate results

■ **Wash hands carefully**
Rationale To avoid contamination and cross infection

■ **Attach sterile needle to syringe/plastic cuff**
Rationale To avoid doing this in front of client and provoking unnecessary anxiety

■ **Approach client, adjust position for procedure**
Rationale To ensure comfort and privacy, ensuring that you will not be inadvertently bumped into

■ **Support the chosen arm and apply tourniquet to mid-upper arm**
Rationale To prevent the arm from moving during procedure. To obstruct venous blood flow, making the veins more prominent

■ **Select suitable vein**
Rationale To use a vein that will maximize successful venepuncture

■ **Open alcohol swab, put on non-sterile gloves and swab client's skin (allow to dry for 30 seconds)**
Rationale To reduce the risk of introducing infection to the woman's circulation following puncture of the skin

■ **Anchor vein with thumb of non-dominant hand**
Rationale To stabilize the vein during venepuncture

■ **Using dominant hand, insert needle into vein, lumen uppermost, at an angle of 30°, until lumen is just no longer visible**
Rationale To enter lumen of vein with needle, with maximum control. To ensure that the needle remains in the lumen, avoiding piercing the other side of the vessel wall

■ **When flash back has been observed, grasp syringe/cuff with non-dominant thumb and index finger, keeping the needle still**
Rationale To ensure needle is in the lumen of vein. To achieve a firm grip on the syringe/cuff avoiding further movement of the needle. The grip may be further secured by wrapping the other three fingers around the client's arm; this is difficult if you have small hands or the woman has a large arm

continued

Box 9.1 continued

- **Use dominant hand to pull steadily back on plunger of syringe or apply blood bottles until required amount of blood withdrawn**
  Rationale To collect appropriate amount of blood with maximum control. Blood bottles should be gently inverted twice, when they have been filled with the required amount of blood in order to mix the blood with the reagents in the bottle

- **Release the tourniquet**
  Rationale To restore the blood flow and reduce discomfort

- **Place cotton wool ball over the puncture site, withdraw the needle completely and apply immediate pressure**
  Rationale To stop the bleeding and avoid bruising at the puncture site. The client can then be asked to continue to press firmly on the cotton wool, thus involving her in her care. She should keep her arm straight, until the bleeding has stopped

- **Label bottles with client's name, date of birth and hospital number**
  Rationale To ensure correct identification of client

- **Inspect puncture site and apply adhesive dressing when bleeding has ceased**
  Rationale To reduce the risk of infection and enhance comfort. Ensure

the client is not allergic to adhesive; if so, a small dry dressing and bandage may be applied

- **Dispose of clinical waste and sharps in line with local policy**
  Rationale To prevent cross infection and needle stick injuries. Each Trust will have a policy for the safe disposal of clinical waste

- **Match blood samples with laboratory request forms and seal in specimen bags**
  Rationale To ensure correct sample goes with correct form and reduce cross infection. Do not wait until the end of a clinic or a batch of specimens as this will increase the risk of identification error

- **Remove gloves and wash hands**
  Rationale To reduce the risk of cross infection and/or contamination

- **Document which bloods have been taken in client's notes**
  Rationale To ensure continuity, completeness and compliance with professional standards

- **Remind client how she will be informed of the results**
  Rationale To involve the client in her care and clarify procedure for receipt of blood results.

1. The midwife discusses the procedure with the woman enabling her to understand its relevance to her care and give consent

It is essential that the woman has sufficient information to enable her to give informed consent for any blood test. The fact that the woman holds her arm out when you sit next to her holding a tourniquet implies that she consents to the procedure. However, it is imperative that the woman knows what her blood is being tested for, not least to avoid embarrassment when results are given, but more importantly, to avoid the possibility of a breakdown of trust that may occur when information is withheld. She may have firm views about certain screening tests, for example, and would have grounds for complaint if a test were performed without her knowledge. Hence the woman should be given the opportunity to ask questions in relation to the blood test and the student midwife should refer any uncertainty to a registered midwife. The woman must understand the implications of the results of the test.

2. The observation is made at the appropriate time according to the woman's plan of care

Local trust policies will provide guidance with regard to when routine blood tests should be offered to women during pregnancy and postnatally. It will sometimes be necessary to adapt this routine plan to respond to the woman's individual needs. For example, a woman who complains of excessive tiredness, faintness and or pallor during pregnancy may have become anaemic. The midwife may therefore decide to take blood for a full blood count even if the booking blood values were within normal range. Whenever a blood test is taken, there should be a plan in place for the woman to receive her results. So, for example, the woman who has presented with possible anaemia may need treatment which should be started as soon as possible to enable her to regain optimum health. All blood results received from the laboratory should be seen and signed by a practitioner and followed up where necessary. Where a blood test forms part of an individual plan of care this should be clearly documented and evaluated.

Activity

Find out what happens to blood results where you work. How are abnormal results dealt with? Whose responsibility is it to ensure that the woman receives the appropriate treatment?

3. The observation is made using the correct technique

The technique for taking blood is described in detail in Box 9.1. As a student you will work with many different practitioners, each adapting the basic procedure to the situation they are in. The way they do things may also reflect the way they were taught and may have remained unchanged since then. For example, some midwives do not wear gloves to take blood, saying that they make them clumsy or it presents the wrong image to women. Make sure that you learn from the outset how to handle phlebotomy equipment whilst wearing gloves. Women expect health professionals to take the necessary precautions to protect themselves from infection and do not want to see you cut corners in any aspect of your care. Modern practice should reflect the philosophy of client involvement combined with scrupulous infection control precautions. Do not compromise your standards – remember you can also be a role model, exhibiting exemplary clinical practice.

Venepuncture is an important aspect of care during the childbirth continuum and any difficulty obtaining the specimen should be discussed with a registered midwife. No more than two attempts should be made. Where a suitable vein cannot be identified, the procedure should not be attempted but referred to a senior colleague.

4. The woman is supported during the observation and her reaction observed

No one likes having blood taken but some dislike it more than others. The student should ascertain whether or not the woman has had blood taken before and how she feels about the procedure. It is not unusual for a woman to feel faint during or after venepuncture. If there is a likelihood of this happening based on the woman's previous experience, it is recommended that she lies down for the procedure, with a left lateral wedge to avoid venacaval compression. There should be no unnecessary delay that could further fuel anxiety. Observing a faint for the first time can be alarming for a student. The main concern regarding the client is that she does not fall off the chair and injure herself and that her airway is patent. The woman who feels faint should be encouraged to lower her head. She should not be left alone until she feels well again.

5. The woman is made comfortable after the procedure

The woman should be informed that the procedure is over and assisted to re-arrange her clothes if necessary. She should sit quietly while the midwife labels the bottles and completes the test request forms, and advised not to stand up quickly, to avoid fainting.

Activity

What does 'syncope' mean? Find out when specimens are routinely collected where you work. How is an urgent specimen transported and examined?

6. The woman is informed of the result

Routine specimens are sent to the appropriate laboratory. Results may take several days to return to the place they were taken, in written form. Many hospitals have electronic systems that enable practitioners to find results via the computer system (password protected) within hours of their being processed. Urgent results are phoned through to the ward or surgery. It is essential that they are recorded accurately and if the student answers the phone s/he should repeat what s/he hears back to the laboratory officer, to confirm that she has heard correctly. The results should then be brought to the attention of the midwife responsible for the woman's care and recorded in her notes. Subsequent action should also be documented and the results discussed with the woman.

7. If the result is outside normal parameters it is reported to an appropriate member of the team

The registered midwife will report any abnormal blood results to a medical practitioner and document that she has done so in the woman's notes. The doctor will discuss a plan of action with the midwife and woman which should then be implemented and evaluated accordingly.

8. An accurate and legible record is made of the observation

When a blood test has been taken this should be recorded in the woman's notes. Any further action regarding follow-up of results should also be communicated to the woman and documented.

Reflection on trigger scenario

Look back at the trigger at the beginning of this chapter.

Emily blinked to find the student peering over her. It was impossible to tell who was the most pale. 'You fainted', the student explained, looking as though she might do the same. 'Oh, I always do that when I have blood taken', Emily whispered, taking a sip from the water that had been thrust into her hand. 'I should have warned you.'

It described a situation in which a woman, Emily, fainted during venepuncture. This could have happened at any point during pregnancy, childbirth or in the postnatal period and highlights physiological, social and psychological issues in relation to this procedure. The jigsaw model will be used to consider the issues in more depth.

Effective communication

Before any procedure is conducted in maternity care, it should be discussed with the woman. It is evident that the student midwife and Emily had not discussed whether Emily was usually alright having blood taken. If it had been ascertained that Emily usually fainted during this procedure then she could have been asked to lie down and the faint could have been avoided. How can this situation be avoided in the future? Is there anywhere in the woman's records where special instructions can be documented?

Woman-centred care

Involving women in their care is central to the provision of individualized maternity care. Women know their bodies and their responses better than

professionals and should be consulted to provide valuable information about how they react in particular situations. Similarly, Emily could be consulted about how long it usually takes her to recover following a faint and what helps her feel better. With regard to receiving the results of her blood test, Emily should be informed of the usual way that results are provided in this situation and asked if this fits in with her. For example, if results are normally posted one week later and Emily is actually going on holiday in a week for a fortnight, an alternative means of communication should be agreed to enable any necessary treatment to be commenced without delay. Woman-centred care is enhanced by meticulous documentation of all care plans. What means of communication have you observed that enhance client involvement in their care?

Using best evidence

There are many examples of how evidence can inform the care of women prior to and following venepuncture. Find the evidence about the best way to provide women with information about antenatal screening. What is the evidence to support the use of alcohol swabs prior to piercing a vein? What research informs the midwife's care of women receiving results from antenatal screening tests?

Professional and legal issues

Midwifery practice is supported by professional guidance and English law that underpins it. For example the Nursing and Midwifery Council's code of professional conduct (NMC 2008:02) states:

You must respect and support people's rights to accept or decline treatment and care.

This means that a woman can refuse to have blood tests taken even if this puts her health or that of her fetus at risk. Reflect on an occasion when a woman refused a blood test. How did the professional react? What documentation was made? Were the woman's wishes respected?

Team working

This scenario highlights the need for professionals involved in maternity care to work together to help prevent adverse incidents from being repeated. The most important feature of effective team working is clear channels of communication, particularly documentation. Systems also need to be in place to summon help should this be required, thus avoiding leaving the woman alone. Can you remember the emergency numbers used where you work to summon medical aid? How do you summon another midwife in an emergency?

Clinical dexterity

Taking blood requires a high level of dexterity that can only be developed through practice and experience. Not only does the practitioner need to be able to perform the task in hand, but also needs to be able to monitor the woman's condition and provide verbal reassurance simultaneously. Have you observed a health professional having difficulty obtaining a specimen? What did they say to the woman? How was the specimen ultimately obtained?

Models of care

If Emily's maternity care was provided within a model that provided high levels of continuity, for example, caseload midwifery, it is probable that her reaction to venepuncture would be remembered by her primary carer and she would be less likely to have blood taken again in a sitting position. That this cannot be guaranteed or assumed means that meticulous documentation becomes even more paramount as it is likely that Emily will meet a range of professionals throughout her pregnancy and labour journey. What other advantages might you expect with regard to venepuncture and continuity of carer?

Safe environment

Taking blood is a potentially hazardous procedure and every care needs to be taken to create an environment that is calm and away from the main traffic of the clinic or ward. Contaminated needles must be disposed of in a sharps bin close to where the procedure takes place to avoid their unnecessary transportation. Care must also be taken to ensure that the blood samples that are taken are stored in a place where they will be collected without undue delay or that appropriate arrangements are made for their refrigeration until they can be safely delivered to the laboratory. What systems are in place where you work to ensure that specimens are collected for transportation to the laboratory?

Promotes health

When the student has become proficient at taking blood and being able to converse at the same time, s/he can use the time to distract the woman by providing her with useful information appropriate to the test. For example, she might explore ways that the woman could increase the iron content of her diet. What advice would you give to a woman regarding an iron rich diet? What information would you need in order to provide this advice?

Further scenarios

The following scenarios enable you to consider how specific situations influence the care the midwife provides. Use the jigsaw model to explore the issues raised in each scenario.

Scenario 1

Julie is pregnant for the first time and goes to see the midwife Alison for some blood tests. Alison is talking her through what each test is for and starts describing the screening test for Down's syndrome. Julie interrupts her saying, 'I don't want that test, my sister has Down's syndrome.'

Practice point

Although the majority of women agree to antenatal screening tests some women have specific reasons why they do not wish to be screened. Midwives have a responsibility to ensure that women understand what the test can offer but should not coerce them or make them feel guilty about their decision.

Questions raised by Scenario 1 include:

- Should Alison continue explaining the screening test?
- What would you say to encourage Julie to explore her feelings?
- Should Julie's partner have any say in the matter?
- What other factors might influence whether or not a woman accepts a screening test?
- Do screening tests diagnose disease?
- Does Julie have the right to refuse the test? What about the rights of her unborn baby?
- What are your own feelings about screening for fetal abnormality?

Scenario 2

Raquel is seeing the last woman in a busy antenatal clinic. 'You are looking rather pale and tired. How are you feeling?' she asks the young mother. 'Yes, I am really tired', she admits. Raquel writes out a form and gives it to the woman, saying, 'Make an appointment at the desk for this blood test as soon as you can.'

Practice point

Women feel tired during pregnancy for a range of reasons and these should be explored before blood tests are requested. Busy clinics sometimes make it difficult to explore all issues in depth, but it may be possible to arrange to see women with particular health needs outside the clinic schedule.

Questions raised by Scenario 2 include:

- What blood test(s) might she be requesting? What is the normal range for this test(s)?
- Why did not she take the test herself?
- Who else is qualified to take blood?
- How would Raquel get to know what the result was? What systems are in place where you work for abnormal results to be followed up?
- Did the woman know what the test was for?
- What might the implications be if the woman forgot to get the test?

Conclusion

Venepuncture is an important aspect of the midwife's role enabling blood to be analysed, providing valuable information about the woman's current health status. It takes considerable dexterity and confidence to master. The student midwife must be able to identify when venepuncture is indicated, how it fits the plan of care and consider how the results will be managed. The woman

must remain central to the procedure, with information regarding specific blood tests not only provided but also interpreted.

Useful resources

http://www.studentmidwife.net/midwifery_resource_videos/348_venepuncture_video.html

References

Beyea S, Nicholl L 1996 Back to basics. Administering intramuscular injections the right way. American Journal of Nursing 6(1): 34–35

Johnson R, Taylor W 2006 Skills for midwifery practice, 2nd edn. Elsevier, Edinburgh

Nursing and Midwifery Council (NMC) 2004 Midwives rules and standards. NMC, London

Nursing and Midwifery Council (NMC) 2008 The Code. Standards of conduct, performance and ethics for nurses and midwives. NMC, London

Rankin J 2005 The cardiovascular system. In: Staples D, Rankin J (eds) Physiology in childbearing with anatomy and related biosciences. Elsevier, London

Stables D, Rankin J 2005 Physiology in childbearing with anatomy and related biosciences. Elsevier, Edinburgh

Chapter 10

Neonatal blood tests

Introduction

There are a number of reasons why a midwife might need to perform blood tests on a newborn baby, and these include: newborn screening tests; serum bilirubin tests; and blood glucose monitoring. All of these tests involve a 'heel prick' to draw a small amount of blood from the baby's heel. This procedure often raises anxiety in the parents and the student midwife in particular. Learning to undertake this test with compassion and dexterity is paramount to minimize the dread it has the potential to evoke.

Trigger scenario

Consider the following scenario and the questions which follow it in relation to newborn screening tests:

Megan, student midwife, felt nervous as she cuddled the week-old baby. Her face was flushed as she turned to the new mother and mumbled, 'You can leave the room while I do this if you want.' She wished everyone would go, including the midwife. Last time she had tried to do the blood spot test, the midwife had to take over. She really did not want to fail again.

What do you need to know in order to interpret this situation? Reflecting on this scenario you may have asked yourself:

- Why would the woman wish to leave the room?
- Why was the student so anxious?
- What was the test for?
- How was it taken?
- Why would the midwife have to take over?
- What could the student do to increase her chances of success this time?

Newborn screening tests

The detection of abnormal conditions in both the mother and baby is an important part of the role of the midwife, as is the ability to recognize when to take action following the discovery of any abnormality (NMC 2004). Screening has become a complex issue as more screening tests become available. The United Kingdom (UK)

National Screening Committee defines screening as:

Screening is a public health service in which members of a defined population, who do not necessarily perceive they are at risk of, or are already affected by a disease or its complications, are asked a question or offered a test, to identify those individuals who are more likely to be helped than harmed by further tests or treatment to reduce the risk of a disease or its complications.

(UKNSPC 2007)

Activity

Consider this definition of screening and reflect upon how women are offered screening in your experience.

Much of the examination carried out on babies during their first year of life is a form of screening, including the newborn examination carried out in the first 24–48 hours of life, and the weight and growth checks carried out by midwives and health visitors. While some tests focus on confirming normality, some tests are carried out specifically to identify certain diseases or conditions. The metabolic screening or dry spot test (also known as the Guthrie test) is one form of screening which tests for certain inherited diseases. The UK Newborn Screening Centre has been set up to monitor this screening programme. Each year approximately 250 babies with phenylketonuria (PKU) or congenital hypothyroidism (CHT) are identified through screening, allowing effective treatments to be started before irreversible neurological damage has occurred, preventing lifelong disability (UKNSPC 2007).

Activity

Name three other screening tests carried out on newborn babies during the postnatal period.

Current metabolic screening (dry spot; blood spot)

Based on the Guthrie test which was developed by Dr Guthrie in the early 1960s, its primary purpose was to monitor blood phenylalanine levels in patients with PKU. It has been used in the UK to screen newborn babies for PKU since 1969 (UKNSPC 2007). Since then a number of other screening tests have been added to the screening programme, including congenital hypothyroidism and a range of other conditions. A spot of blood from a heel prick is collected on a piece of blotting paper and allowed to dry. The Guthrie card enables four separate spots of blood to be collected and hence a range of conditions can be identified. Discs of this paper are then punched out and subjected to laboratory testing. This test is usually performed on or around the sixth postnatal day.

The conditions that are screened for may vary between health authorities. Cystic fibrosis screening is currently being implemented across England but is still not available in all areas (UKNSPC 2007).

Some health authorities undertake anonymous HIV prevalence surveillance using the Guthrie card. The midwife must keep abreast of such developments in order to provide parents with accurate information about the screening of their baby (NMC 2004). It is essential that the practitioner develops an understanding of the conditions that the sample will be tested for so that she can provide parents with accurate information in a clear and concise manner.

Phenylketonuria (PKU)

This is an autosomal recessive condition affecting approximately 1 in 10 000 newborn babies (Hull & Johnston 1993). The enzyme phenylalanine hydrolase is missing from the liver and thus phenylalanine cannot be converted to tyrosine. Phenylketones build up in the blood, accumulate in the brain and result in permanent brain damage (Burroughs & Leifer 2001). However, if detected early, damage can be prevented by the strict application of a phenylalanine-restricted diet.

Capillary blood is collected from the neonate via the Guthrie test. The test involves placing the punched spot of blood-soaked filter paper onto a plate of agar jelly with a bacterium that requires phenylalanine in order to grow. A positive test is therefore one in which the bacteria has grown. Bacterial growth may be inhibited if an alcohol swab is used: they should therefore not be used for Guthrie tests.

The practitioner taking the test must ensure that she documents when the baby had its first milk feed, as the baby must have ingested milk protein for at least 48 hours for a positive result to be obtained (Johnson & Taylor 2006).

If the baby is receiving antibiotics, either directly or via breast milk, they can inhibit growth of the bacteria leading to a false negative result. Johnson & Taylor (2006) recommend taking the test 48 hours after the antibiotic course has been completed.

Congenital hypothyroidism (CHT)

Babies with congenital hypothyroidism do not produce thyroid hormones properly, which can affect the development of the baby's organs, in particular the brain (UKNSPC 2007). If the condition is identified early the baby can be treated and can lead a healthy life (UKNSPC 2007).

Cystic fibrosis (CF)

CF is caused by a genetic defect occurring on the CFTR gene. Many parts of the body are affected including the pancreas and its secretions leading to malabsorption, malnutrition and vitamin E deficiency, and the lungs, resulting in frequent chest infections and lung damage. Cystic fibrosis also causes infertility in males and a shortened life expectancy.

Sickle cell disease (SCD)

SCD is an inherited disorder of the red blood cells which leads to haemolytic anaemia with the blood cells changing into a sickle shape. The sickle cells cause thrombosis and obstruction in small vessels, leading to tissue ischaemia and necrosis. The mutated allele is recessive, meaning it must be inherited from each parent for the individual to have the disease. Screening for sickle cell disease aims to identify affected infants, as early diagnosis allows prophylaxis with penicillin and vaccines, and parent training to identify children with complications and to present early for treatment which has been found to reduce complications and deaths in young infants (NHS Sickle Cell and Thalassaemia Programme 2007).

Medium chain acyl co-A dehydrogenase deficiency (MCADD)

MCADD is a rare hereditary disease that results from the lack of an enzyme required to convert fat to energy. The disease complications usually occur when the baby has long periods between meals, causing the body to use its fat reserves for energy. When this action is blocked by the lack of the necessary enzyme, serious life threatening symptoms and even death can occur. With early detection and monitoring, children diagnosed with MCADD can lead normal lives. All newborns will be screened for MCADD by March 2009 (UKNSPC 2007).

Other neonatal blood tests

Serum bilirubin test (SBR)

In their first few days of life, all babies begin to destroy fetal red blood cells, replacing them with new red blood cells. The rapid destruction of red blood cells and subsequent release of fetal haemoglobin into the bloodstream results in the production of bilirubin, a waste product produced by the

liver. Bilirubin is excreted in bile, and eliminated in the faeces. Immediately after birth, more bilirubin is produced than the infant's immature liver can handle, and the excess remains circulating in the blood. This can lead to neonatal jaundice, which if severe can lead to complications.

> **Activity**
>
> Check that you understand about the complications of hyperbilirubinaemia.
>
> Write down the clinical signs and symptoms of neonatal jaundice.
>
> Check that you understand what is meant by conjugated and unconjugated bilirubin.

The level of bilirubin in the newborn's blood can be measured via the SBR test. The bilirubin test will determine if hyperbilirubinaemia is present and allows the neonatal team to determine if the condition is relatively normal (benign) or possibly related to liver function problems or other conditions.

Blood glucose test (BM)

Glucose is the main energy source for the newborn baby and the brain depends almost exclusively on this energy, but glucose regulation mechanisms are sluggish at birth. This leaves the newborn at risk of hypoglycaemia if metabolic demands are increased or in the presence of other conditions. Severe or prolonged hypoglycaemia can lead to long-term brain damage. Blood glucose can be measured using heel prick blood on a specially designed reagent strip which is then inserted into a glucometer for reading.

Ensure you know what conditions might put babies at risk of low blood glucose.

List the symptoms of low blood glucose.

The procedure for obtaining a heel prick specimen of blood

1. The midwife discusses the procedure with the woman enabling her to understand its relevance to her care and give informed consent

The client should have been given information regarding the screening test prior to the date set for it to be carried out. For the SBR and BM, the client should be fully aware of the nature and reasons for the test and what to expect from you and the other members of the midwifery care team. It is your responsibility to check that the client has had and understood this information, and at the same time you should check the plan of care for any other relevant information. The need to discuss the relative benefits of newborn screening should not be overlooked in your haste to complete the procedure. Similarly, parents need to know what the subsequent actions might be following the BM or SBR test.

Carrying out the 'heel prick' involves balancing the need to collect sufficient blood, with the potential for discomfort for the baby and unease for the parents. The parents should be prepared for what you are going to do and offered the option to leave the room if they feel they will be distressed. However, it may

be useful to perform the procedure with the parent holding the infant.

2. The procedure is carried out at the appropriate time according to the woman's plan of care

The test for phenylketonuria should be carried out on the 5th–8th day postnatally, which means that the whole screening test is carried out at this time. The timing of the procedure should ideally be at the mother's convenience and should only take place once she is ready.

An SBR or BM test should be carried out as described in the infant's care plan. SBRs may be ordered to diagnose neonatal jaundice, and then further carried out at regular intervals to monitor the effectiveness of phototherapy in treating the jaundice. Similarly, BMs may be diagnostic or performed to monitor the baby's condition. BMs may be ordered as pre- and post-feed, and it is essential that the student midwife and the client are aware of these requirements, so that the test is carried out at the correct time.

3. The procedure is carried out using the correct technique

Prior to the procedure, the infant's details should be carefully recorded on the screening card, and checked for accuracy.

Wash hands thoroughly prior to performing the procedure. The site most commonly used for taking capillary blood from a baby is the heel. Care must be taken to avoid the calcaneus (heel bone) and the plantar arteries and nerves in order to avoid infection, haemorrhage or nerve damage. The calcaneus is nearest the skin at the posterior curve of the heel, and this aspect of the heel must therefore be avoided. The only sites for heel prick are the medial or lateral aspects, which are also the furthest away from the arteries and nerves. There should be only one prick of the heel. If another test is required, the other foot should be used. The sterile lancet or autolet used to puncture the skin should only sink to a depth of approximately 2 mm and no more than 2.4 mm (Johnson & Taylor 2006). For a step-by-step procedure see Box 10.1.

To achieve maximum perfusion of the foot, speeding up the procedure, it is worth spending some time preparing the area. Parents can be advised to put socks on the baby the night prior to taking the specimen. The foot can be gently massaged to encourage blood flow and even soaked in warm water if it is obviously cool to the touch.

Box 10.1 Procedure for obtaining a heel prick specimen of blood

- **Consult the client's plan of care**
  Rationale To ensure that the client's condition is monitored effectively. The client should be sufficiently involved in the care of her baby that she is expecting the test to be performed
- **To ensure continuity, completeness and compliance with professional standards.**
  Rationale To ensure that the parent is aware of the nature and purpose of the test and how results are conveyed
- **Assess the possibility of confounding factors**
  Rationale To ensure results reflect true clinical picture
- **Complete the documentation on the Guthrie card**
  Rationale To confirm baby's details with parent
- **SBR and BM – complete infant records**
  Rationale To avoid having to handle the card following the procedure
- **Locate appropriate equipment**
  Rationale To undertake required Guthrie test in efficient manner.
  To avoid having to suspend the procedure due to missing equipment or put baby at risk of delay or discomfort

- **Wash hands**
  Rationale To avoid contamination of Guthrie card. To avoid cross contamination of the infant. To ensure accurate results
- **Provide opportunity for parent to leave the room**
  Rationale To avoid unnecessary anxiety for parent.
  To enable practitioner to focus on care of baby
- **Expose foot of baby and massage gently**
  Rationale To assess appropriate site for heel prick. To achieve optimum perfusion of foot
- **Clean the foot with warm water, dry thoroughly**
  Rationale To avoid the possibility of contamination. To ensure results reflect true clinical picture
- **Apply non-sterile gloves**
  Rationale To protect practitioner from infection risk presented by body fluids
- **Grasp the baby's ankle and flex the foot, using non-dominant hand**
  Rationale To stabilize the foot prior to capillary sampling

continued

Box 10.1 continued

- **Puncture heel with autolet or sterile lancet, using dominant hand. Wipe away first drop of blood with cotton wool**
  Rationale To obtain capillary sample of blood, avoiding contamination
- **Apply blood to Guthrie card**
  Rationale To soak card with required amount of blood
- **SBR – collect blood in capillary tube and cover**
  Rationale To fill tube with sufficient blood and ensure accurate results
- **BM – apply blood to BM stick**
  Rationale To ensure accurate results
- **Apply cotton wool to heel with firm pressure**
  Rationale To achieve haemostasis
- **Apply adhesive dressing**

  Rationale To keep puncture wound clean
- **Dispose of clinical waste and sharps in line with local policy**
  Rationale To avoid risk of needle stick injury. To protect practitioner from infection risk presented by body fluids
- **Remove gloves and wash hands**
  Rationale To reduce the risk of cross infection and/or contamination
- **Inform the parent what happens to the result of the Guthrie test**
  Rationale To involve the client in the care of her baby
- **Document completion of the procedure**
  Rationale To ensure continuity, completeness and compliance with professional standards.

Practise holding a doll on your knee as though you were taking a sample from the right heel, medial aspect. Now try holding the doll as though you were taking a sample from the left heel, lateral aspect. Which feels most comfortable for you?

The heel prick test requires considerable skill and dexterity on the part of the practitioner. Not only does she need to understand the importance of acquiring accurate information for the card itself but she also needs to be able to provide information in such a way that parents understand why the test is being advised. The practitioner must be able to hold the baby safely and calmly whilst at the same time manipulating sharp equipment and the Guthrie card. The heel puncture will be taken from the baby's heel. The foot will then be allowed to hang down to increase the blood flow

and the circles on the blood spot card will be filled completely.

For the SBR, the site is accessed in the same way but the blood is collected in a capillary tube which must be filled to an adequate level for the test to be performed. The sample must be placed in a disposable tray or kidney dish and covered, as sunlight can denature the blood and cause an inaccurate result. The sample is taken immediately to the laboratory or to the neonatal unit for testing.

When performing the BM test, again, blood is drawn by the same method, and the drop of blood is dropped onto the testing strip. The strips should have been checked against the serial number in the machine, and the machine should have been subject to regular quality control checks. This ensures accuracy of readings.

The dry spot test is an important neonatal screening test and any difficulty obtaining the specimen must be discussed with a registered midwife. If the parents refuse to allow the test to be taken, this should be documented in line with local policy and the general practitioner informed.

If the student midwife cannot obtain blood for the SBR and BM tests, it is important that she immediately refers to another midwife or a member of the neonatal team in order to ensure that the tests can be carried out.

4. The baby is supported during the observation and his/her reaction observed

The comfort of the baby should not be compromised during this test and every effort should be made to ensure that the baby is not subject to a prolonged procedure. For this reason, the student midwife can prepare herself in a number of ways, before she attempts to perform the test under the midwife's close supervision. She should observe the procedure until she is familiar with each aspect of it, including documentation, counselling of the parents, preparation of the heel, the heel prick and collection of blood, haemostasis and safe disposal of clinical waste and sharps. It is undue squeezing of the foot that is painful for babies, and this should not be necessary. When the student is first developing the skill of capillary sampling, she may not always be able to collect the specimen without the assistance of the midwife. The need to hand the baby over to the midwife should not be delayed if difficulties are experienced.

The baby should not have an adverse response to the heel prick test. However, the infant must be observed throughout

the procedure and continue to be seen as an individual requiring care rather than a foot that must be made to bleed. It is normal for the baby to cry following the initial puncture of the skin.

5. The baby is made comfortable after the procedure

After the heel prick test is completed, any excess blood from the baby's heel will be wiped away and gentle pressure applied to the wound using a cotton wool ball to prevent excessive bleeding and bruising and to protect the wound. It is important that the baby is not left until the puncture site has stopped bleeding. Mother and baby should be reunited and reassured that the test has been successfully taken.

6. The woman is informed of the result

Woman-centred care means that the parent(s) of the baby should be involved at all stages of the testing process. It is important, therefore, that they are fully informed of the results. Parents will need to know that they will not normally hear about the results of the

Activity

Find out what the normal values are for SBR. Think about the implications of an abnormal result.

Find out the normal blood glucose values. What is the definition of hypoglycaemia in your place of work?

Identify and read the protocols and guidelines which exist for the management of neonatal hypoglycaemia.

dry spot test, but that the results are forwarded to the health visitor.

SBR and BM results should be communicated to the mother of the baby and their significance explained. It is important to refer to the other members of the team who will be involved in care.

7. If the result is outside normal parameters it is reported to an appropriate member of the team

As in Point 5 above, any deviations from the norm should be reported to neonatal or obstetric colleagues, or the GP if the woman is being cared for in the community.

8. An accurate and legible record is made of the procedure

Correct completion of the Guthrie card is essential to ensure that the baby has been correctly identified with information that corresponds to the information provided on the notification of birth. Confounding factors, such as delayed milk ingestion or antibiotic therapy, must also be clearly identified. Many public health laboratories produce self-addressed envelopes for the fast and efficient transportation of Guthrie cards. The midwife must aim to post each specimen on the day it is collected, to avoid delay in treatment of an identified congenital condition.

The SBR or BM should be recorded in the infant's notes and on the appropriate charts. They should also be communicated to the midwife in charge of the case, and to the baby's neonatal SHO or registrar, and this should also be recorded in the notes. It is vital that results are communicated immediately as they directly influence the care of the baby.

9. After use, equipment and materials are cleaned and returned to the correct location for storage, sterilization and transportation, and waste is disposed of in an appropriate safe manner and place

The practitioner must follow universal precautions when dealing with body fluids, to protect both herself and others from cross infection. A sharps box should be used for the disposal of the lancet/autolet.

Reflection on trigger scenario

Reconsider the trigger scenario:

Megan, student midwife, felt nervous as she cuddled the week-old baby. Her face was flushed as she turned to the new mother and mumbled, 'You can leave the room while I do this if you want.' She wished everyone would go, including the midwife. Last time she had tried to do the blood spot test, the midwife had to take over. She really did not want to fail again.

Has this ever happened to you? Now that you have an understanding of the purpose and procedure used for obtaining a heel prick specimen of blood from a baby, the jigsaw model will be used to explore this scenario in more detail.

Effective communication

Having a blood test is a stressful time for any person, and it can be more so for parents to observe their newborn babies undergoing a potentially painful procedure. This means that effective communication is not only vital in preparing the woman and her family for the procedure, but also in ensuring they have understood the reasons for the test.

Verbal and non-verbal communication should always support an open and sensitive approach. Questions which arise from the scenario include: has the woman been prepared for the test? Does she understand its significance, the consequences of the screening? Has the midwife checked that the student midwife has the knowledge and skills required to discuss the issues sensitively with the client? Were the informational materials given to the woman appropriate for her?

Woman-centred care

The provision of sensitive and supportive care means that the woman should feel involved at every stage of the process. However, it might be that the woman also feels the need to leave the room when the baby is undergoing the procedure, and this should also be supported. A professional, caring attitude should allow the woman to make this choice and be able to trust that those caring for the baby will carry out the procedure as painlessly as possible. Questions to ask include: how has the student involved the client in the care up to this point? Has she taken into account any other factors which might affect this situation? What factors in the woman's social and medical history might impact on the screening test procedure or consequences?

Using best evidence

To provide the best standard of care in this instance, the student midwife must utilize the best procedure for obtaining and collecting the blood, and must also ensure the protocols for testing and sending the specimens are closely followed. Questions that may arise include: How has blood been drawn from the heel? There are newborn automated devices and single lancets available. Which of these are most effective? What are the local guidelines for this procedure? Where can I access the latest evidence around screening tests?

Professional and legal issues

Midwives are regulated by law and by a central professional body to ensure the highest standard of care is provided across every situation. In order to explore this scenario further, you might want to ask: What rules or guidelines govern the provision of newborn screening? What aspects of the Midwives' Rules and Code of Conduct apply to this situation? How can midwives ensure they gain true informed consent for the procedure? What would the role of the midwife be if the result was abnormal?

Team working

Midwives are autonomous practitioners within a defined sphere of practice, but are a vital part of a wider team providing care to mother, infant and family. Questions that may arise include: Who might take the blood if the student midwife is unable to do so effectively? While a midwife takes the blood, others test it, record the results and communicate those results to the appropriate people. Who else might be involved in the screening process? And who else might be involved if there was a 'positive' result?

Clinical dexterity

This is a vital part of appearing competent and confident with the procedure, which ensures it is effective and also instils confidence in the client. The student should be familiar with and comfortable with the equipment. Questions include: How can the student midwife develop the dexterity to perform this procedure on a wriggling, crying baby? What equipment is involved in neonatal blood tests? How can the student midwife practise the procedure in other ways? What other factors in their approach, manner and practice can support them to develop this skill?

Safe environment

Midwives must provide care in a variety of situations and environments. The newborn screening typically takes place in the client's home. Questions include: Is there somewhere to wash hands? How will the sharps and waste be disposed of? Is the room set up to allow the midwife to perform the blood test safely, with the space to access the baby comfortably? What risks are involved in this procedure? What risks are there in the environment?

Promotes health

The provision of screening can be viewed as an act of health promotion in itself, but there are other questions to be raised: Will the test harm the baby? What opportunities exist in this situation to educate, inform and support parents about health promotion and infant health?

Further scenarios

The following scenarios enable you to consider how specific situations influence the care the midwife provides. Use the jigsaw model to explore the issues raised in each scenario.

Scenario 1

Gemma is 19 years old, and has given birth to a baby girl two days ago. You have noticed the infant is jaundiced, reported it to the midwife in charge, and been asked to carry out an SBR on the baby. You collect the equipment needed, explain the test to Gemma, and proceed to carry it out, hurrying away afterwards with the capillary tube to take it for testing in the neonatal unit.

Practice point

When considering the need to investigate the severity of observed neonatal jaundice it is important to consider the baby as a whole. If the baby is alert and feeding well and more than 24 hours old, it may be more appropriate to observe the baby over the next 24 hours rather than cause unnecessary anxiety, pain and expense by relying on chemical tests rather than observational skills.

Further questions specific to Scenario 1 include:

- How do you explain the test to Gemma without causing her undue worry about her child's health?
- Why might the midwife have ordered an immediate SBR?
- How can you support Gemma whilst simultaneously ensuring the blood sample is immediately and safely taken for testing?
- How will you record the results, and to whom will you report them?

Scenario 2

You are looking after Suraya, who has gestational diabetes and had a baby yesterday. Her care plan states that the baby must have a pre- and post-feed BM. You come into the room just as Suraya is putting the baby to the breast, and ask if it has had its blood test. Suraya responds saying that she thought the test was only carried out after a feed.

Practice point

It is important that parents receive accurate information regarding tests they or their babies may need. Information given verbally should be further reinforced by a written information leaflet where possible, in the client's first language.

Further questions specific to Scenario 2 include:

- What factors do you think might have affected Suraya's understanding about the BM measurements?
- How can you educate and support Suraya to ensure the BMs are taken at the appropriate times?
- Why does the baby need these BM tests at these times?
- How will you record the results?
- To whom will you refer to report the results and seek input if the results are abnormal?

Useful resources

Cystic fibrosis
http://www.gosh.nhs.uk/newborn/cf/screening/index.htm

National Society for PKU
http://www.nspku.org/

References

Burroughs A, Leifer G 2001 Maternity nursing: an introductory text. WB Saunders Company, Philadelphia

Hull D, Johnston D I 1993 Essential paediatrics, 3rd edn. Churchill Livingstone, Edinburgh

Johnson R, Taylor W 2006 Skills for midwifery practice, 2nd edn. Harcourt Health Science, Edinburgh

NHS Sickle Cell and Thalassaemia Screening Programme 2007. Online.

- What other observations might you make in relation to the baby's condition?

Conclusion

Undertaking the neonatal screening test is an important aspect of the midwife's role. The student will learn to identify when it is indicated and what it tests for, develop the skill of performing it safely and consider how results are managed. Carrying out SBR and BM testing is also a vital aspect of midwifery care of the newborn infant, in identifying any deviations from the normal in order to refer care to the appropriate professional (NMC 2004). The baby and the parents must remain central to these important tests, with information provided in a clear and comprehensible manner, enabling parents to participate actively in the care of their baby.

NHS Sickle Cell & Thalassaemia Screening Programme
http://www.screening.nhs.uk/sicklecellandthalassaemia/index.htm

UK National Screening Programme Centre (2007)
http://www.newbornscreening-bloodspot.org.uk/

Available: http://www.screening.nhs.uk/sicklecellandthalassaemia/index.htm

Nursing and Midwifery Council (NMC) 2004 Midwives rules and standards. Online. Available: www.nmc-uk.org 24 Apr 2007

UK National Screening Programme Centre 2007. Online. Available: http://www.newbornscreening-bloodspot.org.uk/ 24 Apr 2007

Chapter 11

Administration of medicines

Introduction

This chapter outlines the principles of drug administration to adults. You will find the term 'drugs' and 'medicines' used interchangeably. This is a huge topic area, therefore you will be directed to explore some issues in more depth, and find out how to implement the principles described, in midwifery practice. For example, although all midwives can administer pethidine to women in labour, each unit may have developed criteria for its use that relate to who can receive it and when, what dose and how often. Although there are drugs that all midwives can use, each individual Trust will also have particular favourite prescription-only medicines (PoMs) reflecting local guidance.

Trigger scenario

Consider the following in relation to drug administration:

Alison was in established labour. She was planning to use pethidine and was requesting a dose. The student midwife was keen to help and asked the midwife she was working with if she could go and draw up the drug. 'Can I have the keys please?' she asked.

Questions from trigger

What do you need to know in order to interpret this situation? Reflecting on this scenario you may have asked yourself:

- What type of drug is pethidine?
- Where is it kept?
- How is it given?
- Can the student have the keys?
- What alternative pain relief is available in the home setting?
- What other drugs can the community midwife administer?
- Does she need a prescription?
- What is the definition of a prescription?

You will find some of the answers to these questions within the chapter.

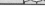

Background

There are fundamental differences between the self-administration of medicines in our own home and the provision of prescribed drugs to clients in our care. Clients place themselves in our trust. If they are in pain, frightened or ill they will often take the medicines we offer or suggest, without question. Our procedures for administration of drugs need to be robust, to ensure that we give the right drugs to the right person at the right time.

Also, when a woman takes two paracetamols at home, she has probably done this on many occasions, throughout her adult life. She knows that she is not allergic to them and that they usually take away her headache. If she is generally fit and well, she probably does not take any prescribed medications on a routine basis, that might react with them. She may also know that if she has just taken a dose, she must wait 4 hours before taking any more.

However, when she comes into the care of maternity services, there are many alternative drugs available. She may take a drug that she has not previously been exposed to and does not know how her body might respond to it. Individuals react differently to the same type and dose of drug. Pethidine is an example of this, with some women feeling little effect and others becoming sedated. She might be offered a drug that could potentially interact with another she has already taken. This will be significant for those women who regularly use 'natural' forms of medicine, such as homeopathic remedies, and midwives should be aware of these women (Tiran 2006). There might be someone else on the ward with the same name with the potential for the wrong drug card to be used for the administration of her drugs.

Between January 2005 and June 2006, 60 000 medication incidents were reported to the National Patient Safety Agency (NPSA 2007), illustrating the need for care in how drugs are administered.

National guidance

Acts of Parliament

There is a detailed legal framework that supports the administration of drugs. The drugs are divided into three categories for the purpose of supply:

- General sales list drugs can be bought without the supervision of a registered pharmacist in a general store
- Pharmacy only drugs must be purchased under the supervision of a pharmacist in a pharmacy
- Prescription only drugs must be obtained by prescription from an eligible practitioner dispensed by a registered pharmacist (Jordan 2002).

Activity

Identify three drugs in each of the above categories. Identify six conditions that can be treated without the need for a prescription.

The legal framework for the supply and administration of medicines is in the Medicines Act 1968 and The Misuse of Drugs Act 1971. The Medicines Act states that prescription only medicines can only be obtained from a registered doctor, dentist or vet. However, midwives have some exemptions from the restrictions in the Act, as some drugs usually available on prescription may be supplied for use in practice, on provision they have notified intention to practice.

The Misuse of Drugs Act 1971 covers the legislation surrounding drugs that may be misused, which are often called 'controlled drugs'. Midwives are included in the amendment to the law of The Misuse of Drugs (Amendment) Regulations 2005 (Statutory Instrument 2005 No. 271) which covers the possession and disposal of drugs. Following the Shipman Inquiry, systems for managing the dispensation of controlled drugs have been strengthened by The Controlled Drugs (Supervision of Management and Use) Regulations (Statutory Instrument 2006 No. 3148) underpinned by the Health Act (2006). These changes are explained in guidance by the Department of Health (2007) and it is now a requirement that Trusts must have an 'Accountable Officer' responsible for managing their safe use and management. It is reinforced that a midwife's records related to the administration of medicines should be audited by their named supervisor of midwives on a regular basis and any concerns reported to the Accountable Officer and the Local Supervising Authority (LSA) Midwifery Officer.

Activity

Find out which prescription only medicines the midwife can administer without a prescription. What drugs do the community midwives carry in your locality?

Patient Group Directions

Patient Group Directions are:

written instructions for the supply or administration of medicines to groups of patients who may not be individually identified before presentation for treatment.

(Department of Health 2000)

This means that there is a detailed document that allows medicines to be given to a particular group of clients, without an individual named prescription. This is particularly useful in the maternity settings as it enables drugs to be given to a woman by midwives, without having to wait for a doctor to physically come and individually prescribe it.

In order to protect the safety of the client and the practice of the midwife, Patient Group Directions (PGDs) are carefully compiled by a multidisciplinary group (Department of Health 2000) and must conform to guidance outlined in the Health Service Circular (HSC 98/051). This HSC summarized the recommendations of A Review Of the Prescribing, Supply and Administration of Medicines under group protocols, the Crown Report (Department of Health 1999) stating that current protocols should be reviewed. Meticulous guidance was given in the Report regarding the criteria for group protocols, under the following headings:

1. Clinical condition or situation to which the protocol applies
2. Characteristics of staff authorized to take responsibility for the supply or administration of medicines under a group protocol
3. Description of treatment available under a group protocol
4. Management and monitoring of group protocols (Department of Health 1999, Appendix A).

In order to ensure that PGDs comply with the law regarding prescription only medicines detailed in the Medicines Act 1968, various Amendment Orders were made which came into force in August

2000, allowing drugs to be administered to an unnamed individual. The exemptions of the Medicines Act (1968) that apply to midwives were unaffected by the new provisions (HSC 2000/026).

Professional guidance

As a registered midwife, you will be personally accountable for your practice (NMC 2004) and this includes the drugs you administer, even though a doctor may have written the prescription. As a student you will be supervised by a registered midwife, who should countersign your records. However, when you qualify, 'you are accountable for your actions and omissions' (NMC 2008:01) and must have an underpinning knowledge of the many different drugs that you will administer to a woman and how they should be given. Following qualification the legislation mentioned in the previous section enables a midwife to supply and give out specific drugs without a prescription, if it is part of their own professional practice (NMC 2007). The Standards for medicines management (NMC 2007) and Standards of proficiency for nurse and midwife prescribers (NMC 2006) cover all the principles in relation to professional practice. Midwives are also accountable for the records that they keep (NMC 2004), including those of the administration of drugs and they are subject to audit by their supervisors of midwives.

Drugs and pregnancy

It is recommended that all drugs should be avoided in early pregnancy if possible and only used if known to be safe during the rest of pregnancy (BNF 2006). As the use of some drugs can result in malformation in the developing fetus, it is essential that caution is used in the prescription of drugs to women of childbearing age. Even if the woman is not thought to be pregnant, but has had unprotected sexual intercourse since her last period, there is a possibility that there may be a vulnerable embryo embedding in the endometrium. Midwives should also be aware that this includes the use of complementary therapies, and women should be advised to avoid their use in pregnancy (NICE 2008).

Activity

If you do not already know its meaning, look up 'teratogenesis'. Find out the name of three drugs that could be harmful during pregnancy.

Drugs and breastfeeding

Care should continue to be taken following the birth of the baby regarding the drugs it may receive via its mother's breast milk. The BNF has a comprehensive section detailing drugs and their use during lactation.

Activity

Identify three drugs that should not be taken during lactation.

Types of drugs

There are many types and forms of medicines and some of their forms of administration are discussed later in this chapter. The issue of injectable forms of medicine will be explored in the next chapter. As indicated previously midwives should also be aware of the use of alternative forms of medicine that may be thought to be innocuous, such as aromatherapy oils , herbal or homeopathic medicine (Tiran 2006).

Controlled drugs

We have used pethidine as an example throughout this chapter. Pethidine is a controlled drug which means that its use is carefully monitored under legislation by the Misuse of Drugs Act 1971. This Act grades drugs according to the harm that their misuse could cause so that penalties can be issued for offences in relation to their abuse.

- Class A drugs include pethidine, morphine and methadone
- Class B drugs include amphetamines, codeine and barbiturates
- Class C drugs include cannabis, anabolic steroids, valium and tranquillizers.

The Misuse of Drugs regulations 1985 categorizes controlled drugs into five schedules (Jordan 2002); see Table 11.1.

Table 11.1 The schedule of drugs

Schedule	Description	Example
1	No health purposes. Possession and supply is prohibited except with Home Office authority. Dose of drug must be in words and figures. Bound register record of supply/administration. Kept in a locked cupboard within a locked cupboard	Lysergic acid (LSD)
2	Opiates and major stimulants. Dispensed on prescription only. Dose of drug must be in words and figures. Bound register record of supply/ administration. Kept in a locked cupboard within a locked cupboard	Pethidine
3	Barbiturates and minor stimulants. Dispensed on prescription only. Dose of drug must be in words and figures. Invoices must be kept for two years	Temazepam
4	Benzodiazepines and anabolic steroids. Not subject to safe custody requirements	Chorionic gonadotrophin (HCG)
5	Weak preparation with little risk of abuse. Not subject to above arrangements. Invoices must be kept for two years	Cough mixtures

As Table 11.1 highlights, controlled drugs such as pethidine have additional controls on the way they are administered. Their individual use is recorded and witnessed by two people, one of whom is a registered midwife or nurse. They are kept in a locked cupboard within a locked cupboard and the keys should be held be a registered midwife. Keys should not be given to other personnel, even doctors.

The administration of drugs

The student midwife should always be supervised when she administers drugs. Some trusts may have local policies regarding the practice of students who are already registered nurses, but care should be taken regarding the interpretation and formulation of such guidance, as the context for the administration of drugs to childbearing women and their babies is complex.

When a student midwife enters the domain of the administration of drugs to clients, s/he must become familiar with a whole new language. There is a plethora of legislation, governmental and professional guidance to understand and apply in practice. The student midwife must ensure that s/he is closely supervised in relation to this aspect of professional and practice development. The principles of drug administration are outlined in Box 11.1.

Midwives should become familiar with how to read a prescription as written on a woman's drug card. One simple definition of prescription is: a written authorization for the supply of a medicine (Department of Health 2000).

It is essential that women understand why a drug has been prescribed. She should be aware of the risks and benefits of her treatment to enable her to provide consent. For most medicines used in midwifery practice, consent is obtained verbally. When confirming the identity of an individual it is good practice to ask them for information, such as 'What is your name?' and 'What is your date of birth?' rather than saying, 'Is your name Lucy Locket?' – clients may say yes in order to comply. Identity should be confirmed with the use of a hospital number on the drug card and wrist label if worn.

In professional practice, you may hear the term 'written up for' meaning that a drug has been prescribed on the client's drug card. It should clearly state the:

- Name of the drug
- Dose (how much)
- Route of administration
- Frequency (how often)
- Special instructions
- Start date
- Signature.

Each of the above is now examined in turn.

Name of drug

Each drug has more than one name. It has a drug or approved name, printed in block capitals in the British National Formulary (BNF). Then there is the proprietary name, with the name of the manufacturer in brackets.

Activity

Find out the approved name for pethidine. What is a proprietary name for oxytocin and who manufactures it? Is Syntometrine an approved name or a proprietary name?

Box 11.1 Procedure for administration of prescribed oral medication

- **Consult the woman's plan of care**
  Rationale To ensure accurate and timely administration of drugs
- **Consult the drug card, identify the drug, dose, route and time of administration, prescriber's signature**
  Rationale To conform with legal requirements and professional guidance
- **Confirm and identify any known allergies**
  Rationale To prevent the risk of allergic reaction in response to contact with known allergens
- **Assess the possibility of confounding factors**
  Rationale To reduce the risk of drug interaction, contraindication, potentiation or overdose
- **Select the correct drug and check the expiry date**
  Rationale To conform with the prescription. To ensure the ingredients are still active
- **Measure the correct dose**
  Rationale To administer prescription
- **Confirm the identity of the client**
  Rationale To avoid giving the drug to the wrong person

- **Gain verbal consent from the client**
  Rationale To involve the client in her care and to notify her of any known potential side effects
- **Observe the client swallow tablets/ medicine**
  Rationale To ensure that they are not left and forgotten, saved until later or consumed by another person
- **Document that the drug has been administered**
  Rationale To ensure that the drug is not inadvertently repeated and to comply with professional standards
- **Evaluate effectiveness of the drug**
  Rationale To ensure that the action of the drug has taken effect
- **Inform medical practitioner if drug has not had the expected therapeutic effect**
  Rationale So that an alternative drug or dose can be considered to maximize client wellbeing
- **Document effectiveness of drug and/ or action taken if drug not effective**
  Rationale To ensure continuity of care through effective communication. To comply with professional standards.

Dose (how much)

Drugs are measured in grams (g) or fractions thereof, and liquids in millilitres (ml).

1 gram = 1000 milligrams (mg)
1 milligram = 1000 micrograms (μg)
1 microgram = 1000 nanograms (ng)

Any quantity less than a milligram should be written in words, as abbreviations can cause confusion, leading to mistakes. Where a dose is not clear or seems unusual, the prescriber should be contacted. The BNF and hospital pharmacy are both invaluable sources of information and should also be consulted if there is any dispute about a dose.

When a liquid is administered, the measuring cup or syringe should be held at eye level to ensure the correct amount is given. Liquids should not be poured back into bottles if the client did not take the drug.

Route of administration

It is vital that the route is clearly identified, as the same dose given by another route can cause serious overdose (for example 100 mg pethidine should be given by intramuscular injection NOT intravenously). The route of administration may be abbreviated:

- p.o. = orally
- p.v. = vaginally
- p.r. = rectally
- i.m. = intramuscular
- s.c. = subcutaneous
- i.v = intravenous

The most common routes of administration are now explored in more detail.

Oral (by mouth)

This is the most common method of administration, the drugs being absorbed into the bloodstream through the walls of the gastrointestinal tract. The rate at which the drug is absorbed will depend on when and in what form it is given. Liquids are absorbed more quickly than tablets, and indeed some tablets are designed to be slow-release. Some women find it hard to swallow tablets and many medications are available through liquid form for this reason. If a drug is taken on an empty stomach, it may be absorbed more rapidly than if taken after a meal. Tablets and capsules should be

swallowed whole unless otherwise stated. When administering tablets, the cap of the bottle is used to shake the required number onto. The tablets are then transferred to a medicine pot before the patient receives them. The practitioner should not handle tablets as she may have a sensitivity or reaction to them.

Sublingual (under the tongue)

Some tablets or sprays contain drugs that are formulated for rapid absorption into the bloodstream, via the rich supply of blood vessels under the tongue.

Injection

This procedure involves inserting a drug directly into the recipient, via needle and syringe. There are three types of injection used by midwives: intramuscular (into the muscle), subcutaneous (under the skin) and intravenous (into a vein). Intravenous injection provides swift administration and a high concentration of drug into the bloodstream, hence smaller does are required by this route (for instructions regarding injection technique, see chapter on 'Administration of injections').

Inhalational

This mode of administration allows a drug that is mixed in a gas and breathed into the lungs, to be absorbed into the bloodstream via the lungs.

Rectal

Drugs designed for administration via the rectum are called suppositories. A drug is inserted into the rectum, where it dissolves. The drugs are absorbed into the blood through the rectal mucosa. Absolute discretion and privacy must be maintained. Following the general principles of drug administration (Box 11.1) the woman should be asked to lie on her left side and draw her knees towards her chest. The practitioner puts on gloves and, using the inside of the packet as a clean field, opens the suppository and applies water-based lubricating jelly to its length. She then washes her hands and applies the gloves. Lifting the woman's right buttock slightly and holding the suppository between her thumb and index finger, the midwife gently inserts the tapered end of the suppository into the rectum. It should be introduced approximately 2 cm beyond the anal sphincter. Any excess jelly is then wiped away and the woman's clothes rearranged.

Vaginal

Drugs designed for administration via the vagina are called pessaries (tablet form). Prostaglandins for the induction of labour are also available in gel form. The student midwife must exercise particular caution when administering drugs via this route, and not step outside the sphere of normal practice. She must be competent in the skill of vaginal examination, be supported by local policy/guidelines and closely supervised. Proficiency at vaginal examination is essential as the prostaglandin is normally placed in the posterior fornix of the cervix, avoiding the cervical os. Normal procedure for vaginal examination and administration of drugs should be followed.

Topical (onto the skin)

Creams and lotions can contain active ingredients for the treatment of many conditions. The instructions must be

followed carefully to ensure effective use, and the stated application should not be exceeded.

Activity

Identify three more routes of administration. Identify a drug commonly used in midwifery practice, for each method of administration.

Frequency (how often)

The frequency of administration must be clearly indicated as again, misinterpretation could lead to either lack of therapeutic effect or overdose. Box 11.2 shows the accepted Latin abbreviations.

Special instructions

Some drugs will require additional instructions for their administration, depending on their action. These may include before food, with food, after food. There may be warnings including: do not drive or operate machinery (if the drug has a sedative effect) or do not stop taking suddenly (steroids need to be gradually reduced) and, commonly, complete the course (antibiotics).

Start date

The start date should be identified on the prescription/drug card. This is important because sometimes a drug is prescribed before it needs to be given, e.g. after surgery.

Signature

Drugs should not be administered without a clear signature on the

Box 11.2 Abbreviations for frequency of administration

Abbreviation	Meaning
o.d. (omni die)	Once a day
b.d. (bis die)	Twice a day
t.d.s. (ter die sumendus)	Three times a day
q.d.s. (quater die sumendus)	Four times a day
o.n. (omni nocte)	At night
o.m. (omni mane)	In the morning
p.r.n. (pro re nata)	When necessary
Stat	Immediately

prescription. The prescriber should state their designation and ideally their bleep number. All instructions should be written in ink and easily read. If there is any concern about interpreting a prescription, its author should be contacted.

Activity

Find out what an unlicensed drug is. Make a note of special conditions which apply to such a drug.

Equipment

The equipment required for administration will depend on the type of drug and on the way it is to be administered. Plastic medicine pots are common, and plastic spoons for oral administration. Syringes and needles will be required for intravenous or intramuscular administration. Different inhalational methods are available. For topical administration gloves may be required, as well as for vaginal or rectal administration; a form of lubrication jelly may also be necessary (see Box 11.1).

1. The midwife discusses the procedure with the woman enabling her to understand its relevance to her care and give consent

It is important for women to understand what drug is being administered and for what reason, prior to her taking it. Communicating effectively with women in this way will mean that they can be more aware of the purpose of the care, but also helps prevent administration errors, as they will be more aware of what they usually take. This is also particularly relevant in relation to drugs administered in labour, so that she may understand what potential side effects may be and enable her to make appropriate choices for her. Further, it will enable her to understand why particular drugs are administered to her baby following birth.

2. The procedure is made at the appropriate time according to the woman's plan of care

Some medicines, such as antibiotics, should be administered at regular intervals in order for them to work effectively. Other drugs, such as controlled drugs, should not be administered too frequently, due to the potential effect on the woman, however ensuring pain relief is given at the appropriate time will enable the woman to either tolerate her pain or be pain free. It is therefore important to know each woman's needs from her plans of care and aim to meet them.

3. The procedure is made using the correct technique

Midwives should be familiar with the drugs commonly used in her place of work, the usual dose of administration and how it is administered. It is also appropriate to know if there are any common reactions between drugs, to prevent administration of these drugs together.

4. The woman is supported during the procedure and her reaction observed

Midwives should be aware of any potential reactions that women may experience on the administration of certain drugs. They should also be aware of those women who may need assistance with taking drugs. Medicines should not be left on the side of lockers to be taken later. Staff should ensure that they are taken at that time or administered later when the woman will take them.

5. The woman is made comfortable after the procedure

After administration of the medicines the midwife should ensure the woman is comfortable, and that she has not had any adverse reactions. Care should be taken to ensure that her dignity is preserved and her clothes rearranged before exposure, following vaginal, rectal or intramuscular routes of administration.

6. Any side effects are reported to an appropriate member of the team

If any adverse reactions to the medicines are noted a medical practitioner should be informed, as should the team leader. Documentation in her notes should be made to ensure that these reactions will be maintained in her records. The woman should also be informed of the reaction so that she may avoid the drug in the future.

7. An accurate and legible record is made of the procedure

The midwife should complete the appropriate chart to show that she has administered the drug to ensure that it is not repeated by mistake. Her signature should be clearly identifiable.

Reflection on trigger scenario

Revisit the trigger scenario from the beginning of the chapter:

Alison was in established labour. She was planning to use pethidine and was requesting a dose. The student midwife was keen to help and asked the midwife she was working with if she could go and draw up the drug. 'Can I have the keys please?' she asked.

The scenario is one that most midwives will come across, that of requirement of pain relief in labour. The storage and administration of pethidine is covered by the legal frameworks described above, especially in relation to the student's role. This chapter has explained some of the legal, practical and professional issues around the administration of all medicines, and should have provided more insight into the issues in the scenario. The jigsaw model will be used to consider the issues in more depth.

Effective communication

The administration of medicines involves appropriate skills of communication, both in the verbal and written form. In this situation the midwife should have built up a relationship with the woman enabling her/him to discuss the different types of pain relief available and to give the woman enough information about them for her to make an informed choice of what is best for her. This is not always easy, however, in the current structures of the maternity services, especially when a woman arrives at a unit in advanced labour. In this situation skills of communication and professional judgement come into play as the midwife assesses whether the woman needs pethidine as the form of relief at the time. Questions that could be asked include: What information has been given to Alison to aid her in her choice? How has she communicated her wishes to the student? Is there a written birth plan? How has the student responded to Alison's request? Where

will the administration of the drug be documented?

Woman-centred care

In this scenario Alison has already indicated her choice would be pethidine for labour. A woman-centred approach may suggest that complying with her wishes is paramount. However, other issues must be weighed up with this request, including the timing of the administration of the drug and the effect on the wellbeing of the mother or the infant. Questions that could be considered include: Is this the best form of pain relief at this time? What alternatives are there for her at this time? Will the administration of the drug promote Alison's wellbeing or cause her harm in the long term? If this is taking place in a home situation will administration of the drug have an effect on her safety in that environment?

Using best evidence

There is evidence available on the effect of pethidine in labour and on how a woman may feel following administration as well as on the effects on the baby (National Collaborating Centre for Women's and Children's Health 2007). The indication is that to prevent accompanying nausea, drugs to help prevent this should also be offered at the same time. Questions that could be asked include: what is the best dose to give to Alison at this stage of the labour? What is the route of administration for the pethidine and the anti-emetic drug? What is the best site of administration?

Professional and legal issues

The legal framework of the administration of medicines is discussed above. Students must follow the rules and protocols of the area in which they are placed and should always be supervised administering drugs, no matter how busy the qualified midwives appear to be. Questions that may arise from this scenario include: Should the student be given the keys? Who should draw up the drug and administer it? Where should the administration of the drug be recorded? On which orders is the midwife acting to be able to give pethidine?

Team working

In this situation the midwife and the student should be working together. It is not clear if this situation is taking place in the woman's home or in a birth centre or hospital environment. There would be team working issues in all these scenarios. If the midwife is busy caring for another woman in labour the student may feel she is trying to take pressure off her by offering to give the pethidine. Questions that arise include: Is there another person the student could ask for assistance? Is there anyone else who could support the midwife if she is not able to give Alison effective support in labour?

Clinical dexterity

When caring for women in labour midwives require ability in clinical skills of supporting the woman and judgement of the best timing and type of pain relief, if required. The procedure for administration of controlled drugs requires practical skills in the drawing up of the medication, usually at speed, as the woman may need the drug urgently. Further, she will need to be able to administer the drug in the correct place when the woman is moving around. A question that could arise is how competent is the student in the

administration of injections? Is she the right person to administer this drug at this time to this woman?

Models of care

In this situation it could be assumed that the student is working in an environment and culture where the use of pethidine is accepted. However, its use has become less common in recent years. Though Alison has made the choice for the use of pethidine in labour it is not clear when and how she came to this decision. Different models of care, such as independent midwifery practice and birth centres, may have different views on the appropriateness of the use and dosage of pethidine in labour. Where midwives caring for women antenatally also provide intrapartum care, they are well placed to understand an individual woman's aspirations for birth and help her fulfil her wishes.

How may these different models affect the use of particular drugs in labour?

Safe environment

The use of a controlled drug is governed by the legal framework already discussed and includes the safety of the environment in which it is kept. Questions that may arise include: Where is the drug kept? How is it labelled? What is the responsibility of the midwife with regard to the keys of the cupboard where these drugs are kept?

Promotes health

In an holistic approach to the promotion of Alison's and her unborn baby's health the midwife needs to consider if the use of pethidine at this stage of her labour is appropriate in the short and long term. Initially, the use of the drug may have a short term effect on helping her through labour, but may make her feel sick or dizzy. Further it may make the establishment of breastfeeding more difficult due to the drowsiness of the baby. By not receiving the pethidine Alison may become more distressed and this may affect her psychologically, causing her to have regretful feelings about her experience of labour. This may in turn affect her long term relationship with her baby. Questions: How can we enable women to make the most appropriate choices for their own wellbeing and for that of their baby?

Further scenarios

The following scenarios enable you to consider how specific situations influence the care the midwife provides. Consider the following in relation to the jigsaw model.

Scenario 1

Krystal has had a caesarean section three days ago. She tells Paula at her postnatal examination that she is feeling very uncomfortable and bloated in her abdomen and she has not opened her bowels since having the operation.

Practice point

Following operative birth many things can affect the motility of the gut: the drugs administered, immobility, lack of a substantial diet, hormonal influences. It is important to assess each woman individually rather than routinely administer drugs to 'solve the problem'.

- What questions should Paula ask of Krystal regarding her diet?
- What suggestions can she make regarding encouraging her bowels to move naturally?

- What medicines may be offered to help relieve the discomfort?
- How are these administered?
- Can Paula administer these on her own judgement?
- Are there any potential side effects to these medicines?

Scenario 2

Wendy is working as a student on an antenatal ward. Jasmeet has been admitted for induction of labour as she is now two weeks past her due date. It is intended that she should be given a prostaglandin in a tablet form.

Practice point

The use of prostaglandins is a common form of induction of labour in women whose pregnancy has gone post-term. The prostaglandin tablets are placed vaginally to enable them to work locally on the cervix and stimulate labour to commence. Midwives should be aware of local Trust policies and procedures concerning the induction of labour.

- What assessments should be made of Jasmeet to establish whether this drug is appropriate for her at this time?
- Have the effects of the drug been appropriately discussed with Jasmeet so that she has been able to make an informed choice?
- Is Wendy able to administer the tablet on her own?
- Does she have an appropriate level of competence?
- Are there any alternative methods or medicines available for induction?
- How and where should the administration be recorded?
- What observations should be carried out following administration?

Conclusion

Even drugs used routinely within the sphere of midwifery practice should only be administered within a framework that protects the woman and the midwife from potential mistakes. Drug errors cause distress and pain for all involved: the application of rigorous systems for the administration of medicines minimizes errors. The student midwife needs to develop an understanding of the drugs used in the care of women and their babies, and ensure that she continues to build on and amend her working knowledge as new drugs and practices come into use.

Useful resources

British National Formulary
http://www.bnf.org/bnf/

The Controlled Drugs (Supervision of Management and Use) Regulations (Statutory Instrument 2006 No. 3148)
http://www.opsi.gov.uk/si/si2006/20063148.htm

Department of Health 2006 Medicines Matter
http://www.dh.gov.uk/en/Publicationsandstatistics/Publications/PublicationsPolicyAndGuidance/DH_064325

Health Act (2006)
http://www.opsi.gov.uk/acts/acts2006/pdf/ukpga_20060028_en.pdf

Medicines Act (1968)
http://www.wipo.int/clea/docs_new/pdf/en/gb/gb091en.pdf

Misuse of Drugs Act 1971
http://www.ukcia.org/pollaw/lawlibrary/misuseofdrugsact1971.html

The Misuse of Drugs (Amendment) Regulations 2005 (Statutory Instrument 2005 No. 271)
http://www.opsi.gov.uk/si/si2005/20050271.htm

National Prescribing Centre
http://www.npc.nhs.uk/

RCM 2006 Midwifery and medicines leglislation: an information paper. RCM, London. Online. Available: http://www.rcm.org.uk/info/docs/Legislation_Info_paper.pdf

RCM Complementary and Alternative Therapies–Guidance Paper No. 6
http://www.rcm.org.uk/info/docs/ComplementaryATguidance_paper_3.pdf

References

BNF 51 2006 British National Formulary. Royal Pharmaceutical Society of Great Britain. British Medical Association, London

Department of Health 1999 Review of prescribing, supply and administration of medicines: final report (Crown Report). Department of Health, London

Department of Health 2000 Health Service Circular 2000/026 Patient Group Directions (England only). NHS Executive, London

Department of Health 2004 Safer management of controlled drugs: the government's response to the Fourth Report of the Shipman Inquiry. The Stationery Office, London

HSC/NHS Executive 2000 Patient group directions (England only). Health Service Circular 2000/026. Online. Available: http://www.dh.gov.uk/en/PublicationsAndStatistics/LettersAndCirculars/HealthServiceCirculars/DH_4004179

Johnson R, Taylor W 2006 Skills for
midwifery practice, 2nd edn. Elsevier,
Edinburgh

Jordan S 2002 Pharmacology for midwives –
the evidence base for safe practice. Palgrave,
Basingstoke

National Collaborating Centre for Women's
and Children's Health 2007 Intrapartum care
of healthy women and their babies during
childbirth. NICE, London

National Institute for Health and Clinical
Excellence (NICE) 2008 Antenatal care:
routine care for the healthy pregnant woman:
Clinical guideline 6. RCOG Press, London

NPSA 2007 Safety in doses: improving
the use of medicines in the NHS. Online.
Available: http://www.npsa.nhs.uk/site/
media/documents/2510_Safety_in_doses_
WEB.pdf 29 Oct 2007

Nursing and Midwifery Council (NMC)
2004 Midwives rules and standards. NMC,
London

Nursing and Midwifery Council (NMC)
2006 Standards of proficiency for nurse and
midwife prescribers. NMC, London

Nursing and Midwifery Council (NMC)
2007 Standards for medicines management.
NMC, London

Nursing and Midwifery Council (NMC)
2008 The Code. Standards of conduct,
performance and ethics for nurses and
midwives. NMC, London

Tiran D 2006 Complementary therapies
in pregnancy: midwives' and obstetricians'
appreciation of risk. Complementary
Therapies in Clinical Practice 12(2):
126–131

Chapter 12

Administration of injections

Introduction

The administration of medications by injection is part of the midwife's role. There may be a variety of reasons for women to need medications given by this route, including the need for pain relief, following the birth of a baby to expedite the third stage of labour, or the giving of Anti D to women who are Rhesus negative. It is important to understand the technique and the procedures involved which ensure safety, accuracy and optimal client wellbeing. It is also important to be aware of the kinds of medications which can be given to pregnant women via this route, and how women may feel about the procedure. Having an injection can be an uncomfortable and stressful experience for women, and so an essential part of midwifery practice is to endeavour to minimize any distress. As a student you must become familiar with the principles of drug administration before you embark on the more advanced skills involved in injection technique, ensuring that you comply with NMC guidance (NMC 2007).

Trigger scenario

Consider the following scenario in relation to drug administration:

Grace was beginning to feel comfortable in the delivery suite environment. She was now in her second year of her midwifery programme and this was her third week on the delivery suite. She felt that she could anticipate what the midwife would do to prepare for the delivery of the baby. Grace was caring for a woman in active labour under close supervision of a registered midwife. When the midwife went to have a quick coffee break the student wanted to show how much she had learned and carefully drew up the Syntocinon, placing it in the receiver on top of the fetal monitor.

What do you need to know in order to interpret this situation? Reflecting on this scenario you may have asked yourself:

- What is Syntocinon used for?
- Where is Syntocinon kept?
- What dose is given?
- Where is it given?

- How is it given?
- What size of needle is used?
- When is Syntocinon given?
- Can a student give Syntocinon?
- Should the student have drawn up the Syntocinon while the midwife was out of the room?
- What rules and guidelines govern the administration of medicines via injection?

This chapter will help you answer these questions.

Background

Administering a drug, by whichever route, is with the ultimate goal of enabling it to reach a target organ or site, in order to achieve a therapeutic effect. Some drugs cannot be taken orally because the acid in the stomach alters their effect, or because they cannot be absorbed into the bloodstream through the intestinal wall. The client's condition may also make the drug difficult to absorb orally. For example, during active labour gastric motility is reduced (drugs are usually absorbed in the small intestine) and a woman's oral intake may be restricted by self-limitations or hospital policy. Some women may feel nauseous in labour. Pain also reduces gastric motility (Jordan 2002) therefore active labour can render the use of oral preparations, requiring systemic action, inappropriate.

Activity

Find out what substances, when ingested, are absorbed directly through the stomach wall.

Injection routes

Drugs are very effectively transported to their target via the vascular system. The speed at which this happens depends on the richness of the blood supply at the site of administration. The route by which a drug is injected must be clearly stated on the prescription chart.

Intramuscular (i.m.)

This is a common route for the administration of drugs in maternity care, including analgesics (pain relief), antiemetics (anti-sickness drugs) and oxytocics (drugs that stimulate uterine contraction). A maximum of 4 ml can be given in a single injection (Johnson & Taylor 2006). In normal circumstances, the drug usually takes minutes to reach the blood supply.

It is important that the site for injection is carefully chosen, to avoid damage to underlying nerves and bone. There are five sites for intramuscular injection (Timby 2005) although the thigh and buttock are the most common.

1. Thigh – into the quadriceps muscle (vastus lateralis) (Fig. 12.1a)

Consider where the arms fall when they hang loosely 'by your side' (you may need to stand up to appreciate this). This is the lateral aspect of the thigh; divide it into thirds, and locate the middle third. This is the intramuscular injection site, and it is particularly useful in midwifery care because it provides easy access for the administration of Syntocinon if

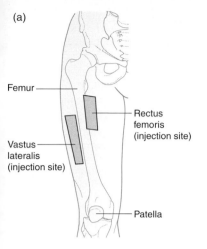

(a)

Femur

Rectus femoris (injection site)

Vastus lateralis (injection site)

Patella

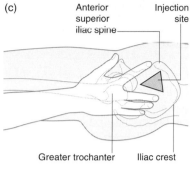

(c)

Anterior superior iliac spine

Injection site

Greater trochanter

Iliac crest

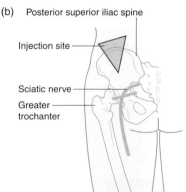

(b) Posterior superior iliac spine

Injection site

Sciatic nerve

Greater trochanter

Fig. 12.1 Sites used for intramuscular injection. (a) Vastus lateralis and rectus femoris sites. (b) Dorsogluteal site. (c) Ventrogluteal site. (Adapted from Rodger, MA and King, L (2000), with permission. Original illustration by Alison Tingle.)

required. It is a suitable injection site for infants.

2. Thigh – into the rectus femoris muscle (Fig. 12.1a)

This site uses the middle third of the anterior aspect of the thigh and is also suitable for infants.

3. Buttock – the dorsogluteal site into the gluteus maximus (Fig. 12.1b)

Imagine someone lying on their front (prone). Looking at a buttock from above, imagine dividing it into four quarters. The injection site is the upper outer quadrant of the buttock. In practical terms, this site can be accessed whilst the woman lies on her side with her upper leg flexed, making her position more stable and the muscle relaxed.

4. Hip – the ventrogluteal site of the gluteus medius and minimus muscles (Fig. 12.1c)

This site is gaining in popularity and can be identified by placing the palm of the hand on the greater trochanter, the index finger on the anterior aspect of the superior iliac spine. Move the middle finger along the iliac crest keeping the index finger in place. The injection site is the centre of the triangle formed between the two fingers (Timby 2005).

5. Upper arm – into the deltoid muscle

This site is rarely used in midwifery practice, but is commonly used for vaccination. It is a smaller muscle and a maximum volume of 1 ml should not be exceeded (Johnson & Taylor 2006). The injection site is the middle of the upper third of the upper arm (outer aspect).

is less vascular, absorption is slower than via the muscular route. This site of injections should be rotated and may be:

> The abdomen
> The outer aspect of the upper arm
> The outer aspect of the thigh.

The technique varies depending on the length of the needle. The needles of pre-packed syringes tend to be shorter and can be administered into the skin (grasped in the non-dominant hand) at an angle of 90°. Longer needles (including the orange 25 gauge needle) should be introduced at a 45° angle. A maximum of 2 ml should be administered via this route (Johnson & Taylor 2006).

Intravenous (i.v.)

This is the site of choice when a drug needs to take rapid effect, for example, during a postpartum haemorrhage. The drug is delivered straight into the circulation and takes effect in seconds. Because the drug is in direct contact with the blood, only small doses of the drug are needed when given intravenously.

Activity

Find out the names of the major nerves that supply the arm, and the buttock/thigh.

Activity

Find out what drug and dose a midwife can give via this route, during a postpartum haemorrhage.

Subcutaneous (s.c.)

This site is commonly used for the administration of insulin or heparin. The drug is introduced between the skin and the muscle and, because the tissue

However, because of the rapid delivery of intravenous drugs and the potential for adverse reaction, this method is not routinely used in midwifery practice. Practitioners who are involved in high dependency obstetric or neonatal care may need to develop competency in the administration of intravenous drugs and should attend a detailed education and training programme in order to acquire and demonstrate this skill in line with professional standards.

Procedure for the administration of a drug by injection

The principle of safe drug administration must be adhered to in order not to put the client at risk. The practitioner must acknowledge the limitations of her knowledge and seek advice where there may be any uncertainty (NMC 2007).

It is good practice when drawing up drugs for injections that two practitioners check the drug together; however, this practice is essential when complex calculations are involved or when controlled drugs are being given (NMC 2007:38). A practitioner must never administer a drug that they did not themselves witness being drawn up. Student midwives should be supervised when they administer injections and have their signatures countersigned by the midwife (NMC 2005:10).

Another cardinal rule is that substances for injections must not be prepared in advance of their immediate use (NMC 2007:28). Although it is tempting to be well prepared for the baby's birth, as in the introductory scenario, childbirth is an unpredictable

process and unanticipated delays are common. Unattended or unidentified drugs are a potential hazard and may be inadvertently and inappropriately administered in an emergency situation.

Equipment

Anticipating an injection is not a pleasant thought and every action should be taken by the midwife to minimize the anxiety women experience before and during the procedure. It is particularly important that all equipment is gathered and prepared out of the woman's sight and that she does not need to be left during the process in order to locate a missing piece of equipment. You will need to locate the drug card, sharps bin and collect the following in a receiver:

Needle, syringe, drug ampoule, cotton wool ball, non-sterile gloves and alcohol swab (depending on local policy).

For step-by-step guide to administration of an injection see Box 12.1.

Needles (Table 12.1)

Needles for the administration of drugs are made in a range of sizes, depending on the route by which the drug is to be injected. They also vary in length and bore size, and are colour-coded for ease of recognition. Needles come in sterile packs and they should remain sheathed prior to use. They are used, not only to administer the drug but also to draw it up into the syringe. Box 12.1 outlines how a drug is extracted from an ampoule. However, some drugs are supplied in a vial with a rubber seal, so that they can be used more than once. To enable the drug to be drawn from the vial, it is easier to

Box 12.1 Procedure for administration of a drug by intramuscular injection

- **Consult the client's plan of care**
  Rationale To ensure accurate and timely administration
- **Consult the drug card, identify the drug, dose, route and time of administration, signature**
  Rationale To conform with legal requirements and professional guidance
- **Confirm and identify any known allergies**
  Rationale To prevent the risk of allergic reaction in response to contact with known allergens
- **Assess the possibility of confounding factors**
  Rationale To reduce the risk of drug interaction, contraindication, potentiation or overdose
- **Select correct drug ampoule and check expiry date of drug**
  Rationale To conform with prescription. To ensure ingredients are still active
- **Select appropriate syringe and needle**
  Rationale To administer the drug into the correct location with the minimum discomfort
- **Gather non-sterile gloves and cotton wool balls in receiver and attach needle to syringe, loosening sheath**
  Rationale To avoid causing undue anxiety to client
- **Holding the ampoule in the non-dominant hand, gently flick the top of the ampoule with the index finger of the dominant hand to expel the solution from the top that will be discarded**
  Rationale To avoid wasting some of the drug or contaminating the environment through spillage

- **Holding the ampoule in the non-dominant hand, firmly snap off the top of the ampoule using the dominant hand and place in receiver**
  Rationale To gain access to the drug
- **Pick up syringe with dominant hand, leaving the loosened sheath in the receiver and invert needle into solution in the ampoule, draw back on plunger with thumb until all solution is in syringe, discard ampoule to receiver**
  Rationale To extract drug from the ampoule
- **Turn syringe, needle uppermost, and hold barrel with non-dominant hand whilst further withdrawing plunger**
  Rationale To ensure all drug now in syringe, not needle
- Holding at eye level, gently tap side of syringe; if air bubbles present, slowly depress plunger until all air is excluded
  Rationale To exclude air from syringe
- **Measure correct dose using divisions on side of syringe**
  Rationale To administer correct dose of prescribed drug
- **Expel any excess into ampoule. Place needle in sheath without touching it**
  Rationale To avoid needle stick injury and keep needle free from contamination
- **Confirm the identity of the client**
  Rationale To avoid giving the drug to the wrong person
- **Gain verbal consent from client**
  Rationale To involve the woman in her care and notify her of any known potential side effects from the drug

continued

Box 12.1 continued

- **Close curtains around the bed, give any visitors the opportunity to leave**
  Rationale To maintain privacy and dignity. To avoid embarrassment or anxiety
- **Locate and expose appropriate site for administration**
  Rationale To gain access to the skin for the accurate assessment and preparation of the site
- **Prepare skin in line with local policy**
  Rationale To avoid introducing infection
- **Put on non-sterile gloves**
  Rationale To protect yourself from contamination with blood
- **Puncture the skin with a dart-like action**
  Rationale To administer drug to client.
- **Withdraw plunger slightly to observe for blood. If none seen, depress plunger with steady smooth action**
  Rationale To ensure that the needle is not in a blood vessel
- **Withdraw needle and cover puncture site with a cotton wool ball applying firm pressure**

- *Rationale* To prevent bleeding from puncture site
- **Assist client to rearrange their clothes and assume dignified position before opening curtains or door**
  Rationale To maintain client dignity
- **Document that the drug has been administered**
  Rationale To ensure that administration is not inadvertently repeated and to comply with professional standards
- **Evaluate effectiveness of the drug**
  Rationale To ensure that the action of the drug has taken effect
- **Inform medical practitioner if drug has not had the expected therapeutic effect**
  Rationale So that an alternative drug or dose can be considered
- **Document effectiveness of drug and/ or action taken if drug not effective**
  Rationale To ensure continuity of care through effective communication. To comply with professional standards.

Table 12.1 Needles (adults)

Size	Colour	Route
21	Green	IM/IV
23	Blue	IM/IV
25	Orange	Sc

by an appropriately trained and competent practitioner.

It has been suggested that a dry needle may minimize pain (Beyea & Nicoll 1996); however, a caring manner and confident technique will help alleviate anxiety and reduce the fear associated with injections.

obtain against suction pressure, if air is injected into the container first. Many practitioners change the needle prior to administration of the drug (Engstrom et al 2000). Intravenous drugs should ideally be given via a cannula, inserted

Activity

Find out the difference between a needle and a cannula.

Syringes

It is important that you select the syringe that approximates to the dose of drug to be administered. To use an over-large syringe would be a waste of resources and it would also exert an undue amount of pressure or suction to the muscle or skin. In most cases in midwifery care, a 2 ml syringe is appropriate for intramuscular injections. When drugs are administered via the subcutaneous route, they often have specific administration equipment. For example, insulin is often given by a pen type syringe, specifically designed for this purpose. Heparin, used for prophylaxis of deep vein thrombosis, is available in pre-packed syringes as the small amounts that are required are difficult to measure accurately.

Activity

If heparin is available in solution 25 000 units per ml and a woman is prescribed a dose of 5000 units, how many ml would be required?

Sharps box

Sharps boxes come in many shapes and sizes and are an essential piece of equipment in the clinical environment. Following use, a needle and syringe should be immediately posted into a sharps box. Care must be taken not to overfill the sharps box as jamming needles into a fixed space could result in a needle being forced through the wall of the box or the hand slipping into the box and a needle stick injury being sustained. Most boxes have a slot at the inside of the posting hole that enables the practitioner to remove the needle

prior to discarding the syringe. On no account should a needle be re-sheathed with the needle in one hand and the sheath in the other, hoping that the two will re-unite. A used needle is a deadly weapon and should be handled very carefully, not forgotten or abandoned, even in the stress of emergency situations. The needle can, of course, be placed inside its sheath following use, simply by locating the sheath in the receiver using one steady hand and not attempting to pick up the sheath until the needle is snug within it.

Activity

Find out what action should be taken in the event of a needle stick injury, in accordance with local hospital policy.

1. The midwife discusses the procedure with the woman enabling her to understand its relevance to her care and give consent

The midwife should explain the need for the medication to be given, the fact that it is to be given by injection, and the site of administration. She should also discuss the effects and side effects of the medication: for example, pethidine can cause drowsiness, hallucinations and nausea and vomiting. Women may ask questions such as: how long will it take to work? Will it be effective? Is there another option to having an injection?

2. The procedure is carried out at the appropriate time according to the woman's plan of care

All medication should be prescribed on a prescription chart, with the route, dose, and time for administration clearly noted. The following guidelines should be observed: Medications should be given at the times stated, and not given more frequently than this in order to avoid overdosing the client. When medications are given by standing order, the midwife must record this in the client notes and on the medication chart. Where a patient group directive or standing order does not exist for a medication, then the prescription must be signed by a doctor and be consistent with the care plan.

3. The procedure is made using the correct technique

The technique for injection is described in Box 12.1. Any member of staff carrying out this procedure should have a good understanding of the technique and, in the case of students, should be fully supervised. The safety and practical points discussed above should be followed.

Activity

Find out what is meant by the Z-track technique for injection and when it is used.

4. The woman is supported during the procedure and her reaction observed

As already stated, this can be an uncomfortable procedure, unpleasant, painful and stressful for the woman. Therefore, it is vital that the woman is made comfortable. She may respond in a number of ways to the injection, and may feel faint. Therefore, it is best that she is seated or semi-recumbent for the procedure, and that she is able to expose the injection site comfortably,

with her dignity being maintained at all times.

5. The woman is made comfortable after the procedure

The woman should be allowed enough time to 'recover' from having an injection, and observed (subtly) for any side effects, such as feeling faint. She should be helped to 'cover up' if necessary, and assisted into a comfortable position for as long as necessary. If pethidine is being administered, or any other narcotic, she should be warned about dizziness and light-headedness and advised to rest until such effects wear off.

6. Any side effects are reported to an appropriate member of the team

Any side effects of the medication or the procedure (such as abnormal bleeding or bruising around the injection site), should be documented and reported to the obstetric team or general practitioner.

7. An accurate and legible record is made of the procedure

Any injection should be fully documented in the woman's maternity notes, care plan or pathway, and medication chart. The procedure should be described, the time and date should be recorded along with the route, site, dose and the names of those who checked the medication and administered it. Signatures should be legible. It is also appropriate to record the professional status of the person who administered the drug and the person who checked it. In the case of the administration of drugs to reduce pain or nausea, their effect should be evaluated and documented.

Reflection on trigger scenario

Revisit the trigger scenario from the beginning of the chapter:

Grace was beginning to feel comfortable in the delivery suite environment. She was now in her second year of her midwifery programme and this was her third week on the delivery suite. She felt that she could anticipate what the midwife would do to prepare for the delivery of the baby. Grace was caring for a woman in active labour under close supervision of a registered midwife. When the midwife went to have a quick coffee break the student wanted to show how much she had learned and carefully drew up the Syntocinon, placing it in the receiver on top of the fetal monitor.

 The scenario concerns a student midwife learning the skills of injections who needs to develop a deeper understanding of the implications of the procedure and the safety aspects associated with it. This chapter has explored the practical and professional issues around the administration of injections. The jigsaw model will be used to consider the issues in more depth.

Effective communication

Effective communication underpins the provision of medications and in particular, the administration of injections. The midwife and the student should have developed a good relationship with the client through good communication techniques and a supportive, professional demeanour. However, the questions we can ask in relation to this scenario include: Why does the student feel she can anticipate the

midwife's future actions? Where has communication 'failed' in this situation? What information has not been shared or passed on by the midwife?

Woman-centred care

In relation to woman-centred care, Grace might be considering that by trying to be efficient, she is helping the midwife focus on the woman's needs in labour. Could her time have been better spent with the woman in other ways? What opportunities would this time on a one-to-one level present for Grace in relation to the provision of woman-centred care? Has Grace checked whether the woman wants or requires Syntocinon for the third stage of labour?

Using best evidence

There is ample evidence surrounding the administration of injections, and some of this is summarized above. It is not appropriate for Grace to leave an unlabelled syringe on top of the fetal monitor, where it could be knocked to the ground by the midwife when she enters the room. The midwife will not have observed the drawing up of the medication, and so has not followed the procedural checks appropriate prior to the administration of the injection. What evidence is there of the effectiveness and appropriateness of Syntocinon for the third stage of labour?

Professional and legal issues

Midwives must be aware of the professional and legal framework within which they practice. In terms of administration of injections, midwives must follow protocols, procedural rules, standing orders and prescriptions. Questions that may arise from this scenario are: What are the implications of the midwife leaving the room? What professional and legal issues are raised by Grace preparing the injection independently? Is she acting on standing orders?

Team working

There is a need to work collaboratively and students and their mentors must work in partnership. But this scenario is taking place on a delivery suite, and so there may be other issues around team working. Could Grace have asked another midwife to check the injection while the midwife was on a break?

Clinical dexterity

The procedure for administration of injections requires considerable practical skill in the drawing up of the medication, the identification of the right site on the body, and the administration of the injection itself. Some of these skills can be practised in simulation situations, and the rest under supervision by the midwife. The student has developed some competence and confidence in these skills. What other issues around clinical skill arise from this situation?

Models of care

In this situation, it is important to consider how the model of care of the delivery suite affects Grace's actions here. Grace is apparently assuming that Syntocinon will be administered to the woman under her care, and is anticipating future actions in a potentially task-oriented way. What might have led to her making these assumptions? How might this affect the woman's experience of care, and her choices in labour?

Safe environment

Leaving an unlabelled injection in the clinical situation could be a danger to other professionals in the room, and a potential danger to the patient if the drug has been left too long out of the vial and has denatured, rendering it ineffective. All contaminated sharps must be disposed of in an appropriate sharps bin as soon as possible to avoid possible needle stick injuries.

Promotes health

Promoting health in this situation should be closely related to woman-centred care. On the one hand, Syntocinon is believed to promote health by reducing the risk of postpartum haemorrhage, which is why it is routinely offered even in low-risk labours. On the other, promoting holistic health requires a whole person approach, meaning that it should be up to the client to make the decision in full possession of the facts, preferably prior to labour. This might be an ideal opportunity, if the decision has not been made, to support the client in an informed decision on the use of Syntocinon for the third stage of labour.

Further scenarios

The following scenarios enable you to consider how specific situations influence the care the midwife provides. Use the jigsaw model to explore the issues raised in each scenario.

Scenario 1

Lucy is in labour with her first child, and has been coping well with the pain using Entonox. She now starts to feel she needs more pain relief and asks for pethidine. She is in such pain that she can't seem to stand still long enough for the injection, as the contractions are very close together.

Practice point

The clinical skills of the midwife in administering the injection here involve more than simply locating the right site and injecting the right drug via the appropriate route. Lucy may need more support from the midwife in order to be able to have the pain relief she has requested. Further questions you might ask are:

- With Lucy in such active labour, is pethidine the right choice of medication for her?
- How can you be sure of proper informed consent when she is in such pain and has been using nitrous oxide (Entonox)?
- How can you ensure Lucy can stay still enough to safely administer the injection and ensure she remains in a safe environment following the procedure?

Scenario 2

Surdeep has been admitted at 34 weeks with suspected premature labour. She has been advised to have steroid injections to mature her unborn baby's lungs. Surdeep does not want to have any injections, and is worried about the effects that the medication might have on her own body. Further discussion reveals she is needle phobic.

Practice point

Midwives often have to deal with women who are extremely distressed by difficulties in pregnancy, and who must weigh up the needs of their unborn baby against their own needs, fears or feelings.

- What skills might the midwife need in this situation?
- What guidance might help the midwife here?
- How might woman-centred care be affected here?

Conclusion

The prospect of having an injection is not pleasant, but the midwife can minimize the anxiety associated with this procedure through careful preparation and a calm and confident approach. The midwife must follow safe techniques at all times, to minimize the risks both to herself and to women she cares for. S/he must be familiar with the procedures around preparation and checking and the routes of administration for the drugs she will administer by injection. S/he must also maintain the highest standards of professionalism through woman-centred care, accurate record keeping and ongoing monitoring of her client's condition after the procedure.

Useful resources

Ventrogluteal site for injection
http://www.nursing-standard.co.uk/archives/ns/vol18-25/pdfs/v18n25p3942.pdf

Injection sites for vaccines
http://www.rcn.org.uk/__data/assets/pdf_file/0010/78535/001753.pdf

References

Beyea S, Nicholl L 1996 Back to basics. Administering intramuscular injections the right way. American Journal of Nursing 6(1): 34–35

Engstrom J L, Giglio N et al 2000 Procedures used to prepare and administer intramuscular injections: a study of infertility nurses. Journal of Gynaecology and Neonatal Nursing 29(2): 159–168

Johnson R, Taylor W 2006 Skills for midwifery practice, 2nd edn. Elsevier, Edinburgh

Jordan S 2002 Pharmacology for midwives – the evidence base for safe practice. Palgrave, Basingstoke

Nursing and Midwifery Council (NMC) 2005 Guidelines for records and record keeping. NMC, London

Nursing and Midwifery Council (NMC) 2007 Standards for medicines management. NMC, London

Nursing and Midwifery Council (NMC) 2008 The Code. Standards of conduct, performance and ethics for nurses and midwives. NMC, London

Rodger M A, King L 2000 Drawing up and administering intramuscular injections: a review of the literature. Journal of Advanced Nursing 31(3): 574–582

Timby B 2005 Fundamental nursing skills and concepts, 8th edn. Lippincott, Williams and Wilkins, Philadelphia

Chapter 13

Surgical care

Introduction

Midwives can be involved in the care of pregnant women undergoing surgery for a number of reasons. The most common surgical procedure is a caesarean section, but other surgery can also be necessary including cervical cerclage, perineal repair or manual removal of placenta under anaesthetic. Occasionally pregnant women need to undergo general surgery such as appendicectomy or cholecystectomy and a midwife is required to check that all is well with the pregnancy. The midwife may have a role in preparing the woman before surgery, being with her during the operation and/ or caring for her as she recovers from the anaesthetic. It is therefore vital that every midwife has a full understanding of the procedures and the care needed to support women undergoing surgery.

Trigger scenario

Read the following scenario in relation to birth by caesarean section. Consider what information you need to be able to interpret the situation:

Julie opens her eyes and begins to shake a little, turning towards the sound of the baby crying. She has just been wheeled from theatre into the recovery room, with an intravenous (i.v.) infusion. Her newborn son is tucked into the cot beside the bed. 'Is that it?' she asks, plucking at the hospital gown. 'What happens now?'

Questions from trigger

- Why has Julie begun to shake after having a caesarean section?
- Why is there an i.v. infusion?
- Why is she wearing a hospital gown?
- Why is she in the recovery room?
- How would you answer her question?
- Did she have a birth partner?
- How does she know it is her baby?

You will discover the answers to these questions within this chapter.

Caesarean section

Caesarean section is the surgical delivery of a fetus through a surgical incision in the abdominal wall and uterus. It is an obstetric procedure carried out by a senior obstetrician, while the woman is anaesthetized, usually with a spinal or epidural anaesthetic. General anaesthesia is avoided except in special circumstances such as severe fetal compromise or at the woman's request. In 2004–05 less than 10% of caesareans were conducted under general anaesthetic (The Information Centre 2006). Casearean birth is a relatively common procedure in the United Kingdom: in 2004–05 11% of women had elective surgery and 12% had an emergency procedure (The Information Centre 2006). Indications for elective caesarean section include breech presentation, multiple pregnancy, placenta praevia, and the prevention of mother to child transmission of infections such as HIV (NICE 2004). Emergency caesarean section is classified by four different grades of urgency: immediate threat to the life of the woman or fetus; maternal or fetal compromise which is not immediately life-threatening; no maternal or fetal compromise but needs early delivery; and delivery timed to suit woman or staff (NICE 2004).

Surgical care

Surgical care involves much more than the provision of care during an operation. It is an holistic process which involves the preoperative period through to the postoperative period, and midwives are involved in every aspect of this care.

Preoperative care

This refers to the care given prior to the surgical procedure. It has also been described as the psychological and physical preparation and assessment of a patient before surgery (Mallet & Dougherty 2000).

Most maternity units will have standard protocols or guidelines which govern surgical care, and within this should be a care pathway for preoperative management. A component of this is the pre-op checklist which records the care given ensuring that all criteria are met for a safe, correct and woman-centred procedure.

Activity

Find out what protocols your unit has for preoperative (pre-op) care.

Find out what pre-op checklist is used in your unit.

Activity

Find out about Mendelson's syndrome and the action which can be taken to minimize the risks. Why are pregnant women more at risk of this condition?

Perioperative care

It is common for the midwife looking after the woman to provide the preoperative care and to then be present in the operating theatre to assist, receive the baby from the surgeon, and care for mother and baby during and after the operation. Therefore the midwife must understand the principles of asepsis in an operating theatre environment. The aim of the operating theatre is to provide an area free from infectious agents (Mallet & Dougherty 2000). Therefore, all personnel wear clean scrub suits, protective footwear, hats

Box 13.1 Procedure for preoperative care

- **Preoperative fasting**
  Rationale To ensure there are no gastric contents which may be regurgitated and then inhaled when the woman's airway is compromised. Women attending for elective surgery should have fasted for 6 hours prior to the procedure (Mallet & Dougherty 2000)

- **Women are given a hospital gown to wear during the procedure**
  Rationale This is recommended because of the likelihood of clothing coming into contact with blood and body fluids

- **Skin preparation**
  Rationale Because of the location of the caesarean incision at the bikini line, it is necessary to shave an area of approximately 1 to 2 inches across the top of the pubic hair. This should be a dry shave using a new disposable razor, and the woman must have given her consent beforehand. Gloves should be worn. A strip of hypoallergenic tape applied lightly can help to remove all the hair from the area afterwards.

  The skin of the abdomen and all around the incision site will be disinfected just prior to any surgery, usually with a chlorhexidine solution (Mallet & Dougherty 2000)

- **Consent gained by obstetrician**
  Rationale A consent form is used and placed in the woman's notes. This process of information sharing should ensure that the woman is aware of the need for the operation and what it will involve, along with any risks and issues about recovery. This should be checked against her ID band, and double checked prior to surgery. The consent

form should be the end point of the discussion which both informs her and helps to psychologically prepare her for surgery

- **Removal of jewellery**
  Rationale Jewellery can pose a hazard in theatre, particularly when diathermy is being used. Also, there is the possibility that valuable jewellery could be lost in theatre. Jewellery should be removed and either placed in the care of a relative or logged into a locked cupboard by the midwife. This should be recorded in the woman's notes. If the woman wishes to keep her wedding band on, it can be taped with hypoallergenic tape

- **Removal of nail varnish**
  Rationale The nail beds can be observed for oxygenation during surgery, and therefore nail varnish should be removed

- **ID bands – name, date of birth, hospital identification number**
  Rationale The woman may be unconscious or compromised and so correct personal identification is vital

- **Record of drug allergies/sensitivities plus red ID band**
  Rationale Identifying any pre-existing drug allergies or sensitivities ensures the woman is not given one of these accidentally

- **Prosthesis**
  Rationale The presence of any prosthesis, including false teeth, caps or crowns must be noted. False or loose teeth can cause choking or becoming dislodged if the woman needs to be intubated. Prostheses can become

  continued

Box 13.1 continued

detached or lost during surgery. Body piercings should be removed or covered with hypoallergenic tape
- **Documentation**
  Rationale Other preoperative documentation should be checked, such as drug charts and anaesthetic charts – ensuring they are correct, for the correct patient and up to date. It should be recorded in the notes what time the woman was admitted to theatre, who was present, and what preparations have been carried out
- **Psychological preparation**
  Rationale The midwife should keep the woman fully informed of all that is occurring and explain the procedures in advance where possible. It is also useful for the woman and her partner to meet the staff who will be in the operating theatre, prior to the procedure commencing.

and face masks. All those directly involved in the surgery should carry out a 5-minute hand scrub with an antiseptic soap or detergent solution, and wear sterile gowns and gloves (Mallet & Dougherty 2000).

On transfer to the operating theatre, the woman's identity should be checked again and she (and her partner if she is having a caesarean under spinal or epidural) should be given a few minutes, if possible, to get used to the new environment. Communication is important in maintaining a good midwife–mother relationship.

The midwife also needs to ensure she is prepared for the imminent birth of the baby, with a resuscitaire checked and ready, and the requisite paperwork and other items ready to hand. The parents may want their child dressed immediately in their own clothes; if so, these can be taken into theatre in preparation for the birth.

It is important to also remember in the case of caesarean that this is a birth environment, as well as an aseptic, operating room. The woman is undergoing an invasive procedure, but it is also almost time for her baby to be born. Women's own wishes should be respected as much as possible (NICE 2004).

The anaesthetist and ODP will help to position the mother for the anaesthetic, which in most cases will be a spinal anaesthetic. For spinal anaesthesia, the woman will need to be supported into an upright seated position, bending forward, and the midwife can assist with this, by placing a pillow on her lap to help support her abdomen, and talking to her during the procedure. If there is to be a general anaesthetic, the partner cannot usually be present in theatre.

Once the anaesthetic has taken effect, the woman will need to be catheterized because the anaesthetic block interferes with normal bladder function (NICE 2004). An indwelling Foley catheter is used with a standard drainage bag, inserted using an aseptic technique. Catheterization also ensures that the bladder will be empty during the operation and not obscuring the uterine incision site, thus reducing the risk of bladder trauma.

During the procedure, the mother will be draped so that she cannot see the operation site although some women wish to see their baby born and the possibility of having a low screen should be discussed if required. Following the birth of the baby, the cord is clamped and cut and the baby is handed to the receiving midwife. It is transferred to the waiting resuscitaire, dried, assessed and then wrapped warmly. Providing all is well, the midwife can then take the baby to its mother and father for skin to skin contact. The midwife must then check the placenta and membranes and take cord blood in two heparinized syringes for cord gas analysis.

Postoperative care

The woman will be transferred from theatre into a recovery room for a period of observation. This may be a designated area or back on the delivery suite. The woman will usually be transferred with an intravenous infusion in situ, and with an adhesive dressing on the wound site. If she has had a general anaesthetic, she will have facial oxygen in place. The anaesthetist will hand over care to the recovery room midwife and describe all the procedures and medications the woman has received, and also explain the intravenous infusion regime and discuss analgesia.

Immediate observations of blood pressure, temperature, pulse, respiratory rate, oxygen saturation and general condition should be recorded. She

should be observed on a one-to-one basis until she can maintain her own airway and can communicate (NICE 2004). Vital observations should be recorded regularly. Usually this would be every 5 minutes for 20 minutes, 15 minutes for the first hour, then half-hourly if the woman remains stable, and then hourly until she leaves the recovery room.

Reflection on trigger scenario

Revisit the trigger scenario from the beginning of the chapter:

Julie opens her eyes and begins to shake a little, turning towards the sound of the baby crying. She has just been wheeled from theatre into the recovery room, with an intravenous (i.v.) infusion. Her newborn son is tucked into the cot beside the bed. 'Is that it?' she asks, plucking at the hospital gown. 'What happens now?'

The jigsaw model will be used to explore the issues relating to surgical care in more detail.

Effective communication

Every aspect of perioperative care should be underpinned with good communication. Explanations of procedures, aspects of care, analgesia and the observations you are carrying out can reassure the woman and ensure that she is included in her care. Verbal communication should continue even if the woman has had a general anaesthetic and appears sleepy or unconscious, because she may still be able to hear those around her. Good communication with the woman's partner/support person will ensure their involvement in care and help them to understand what is going on and why.

Keeping detailed records is also important. Postoperative care planning takes place in the recovery room, usually, and there may be standard care plans or care pathways which should be individualized for the woman and inserted in her records. Any particular needs that this woman has should be included in her care plan. These might include special communication or cultural needs, issues around infant feeding, or social needs.

Woman-centred care

At this time, the woman is in need of total nursing and midwifery care, as she has had major abdominal surgery. She will be in pain due to the wound, will be feeling tired and may present with some symptoms of shock. If the woman has been involved in care planning prior to the operation, she should have to some extent been prepared for some of these symptoms. Pain relief is vital in ensuring this woman can recover and can start to interact with her baby immediately.

Julie will need a lot of re-orientation information and reassurance that the procedure is over and what the outcome was, especially if this was an emergency rather than an elective procedure. She may not have been emotionally prepared for a surgical birth and may need considerable support in adjusting to the nature of her birth experience. If she has had a general anaesthetic, her level of consciousness needs to be monitored.

Comfort is important. The anaesthetic should provide continuing pain relief but there may be the need to administer analgesia in the recovery room. Usually this will be an opiate for severe pain, typically morphine 10 mg intramuscularly, or an intrathecal opiate administered via an epidural catheter. The woman may also be prescribed oral analgesia, which could be a non-steroidal anti-inflammatory drug such as diclofenac, or may have been provided with a patient controlled analgesic (PCA) device. It is important to check the medication chart carefully, as the woman may have been given rectal analgesia in theatre in order to maximize her comfort in the recovery period (NICE 2004).

Activity

Find out what pain relief is prescribed for postoperative pain in your unit.

Find out what the route of administration is for this pain relief, what the side effects are and how it is prescribed.

What are the issues around use of analgesics and breastfeeding?

Women will also feel uncomfortable once their anaesthetic has worn off, perhaps due to a long period of immobility, and also due to bruising of the abdomen from the procedure. You should discuss this with women and consider what can be done to relieve this discomfort. It is vital that the woman has adequate pain relief before she begins to mobilize postoperatively.

Pressure area care is also another aspect of postoperative care that should be considered here. There is a modified Waterlow Score Chart used for assessing pressure sore risk, and this can be used preoperatively to assess risk and postoperatively to reassess the risk of pressure area damage. The woman undergoing caesarean section is at risk of developing pressure sores, particularly of the heels, because epidural anaesthesia produces sensory and motor block, and restricts movement (Shah 2000). Women are encouraged to move and mobilize as soon as possible after caesarean, and this should reduce any risk of pressure area damage.

Some women having undergone this procedure may experience some psychological effects, and it is important to ensure that the woman has every opportunity to discuss how she is feeling, and how she felt during the operation. Her mood and responses should be monitored. Immediate skin to skin contact can be commenced for mother and baby, once the mother has been transferred to the recovery room, and this should be encouraged because it improves maternal perceptions of the baby, mother skills, mothering behaviour, breastfeeding outcomes, and also reduces infant crying (NICE 2004).

If the mother is too tired or uncomfortable, the baby can be put skin to skin with its father or the mother's partner/support person until she is able. Skin to skin contact can encourage early commencement of feeding. The midwife will need to assist the woman into a comfortable position and help with positioning and attachment, using pillows to help the woman find a sustainable position in which to feed the baby. Again, early mobilization encourages the woman to care for her baby as independently as possible, but support and adequate analgesia are vital. Women should be reassured that there is someone to assist them with all the basic aspects of infant care until she is able to do them for herself.

Wound care should commence from the moment the woman is taken to the recovery room, and the wound site and dressing should be checked regularly for any signs of oozing, bleeding, or haematoma formation, which would be characterized by swelling behind and around the wound, redness of the skin, and increased localized tenderness and pain. The wound dressing should be firmly fixed, and stay in situ for 24 hours (Boyle 2006). If there is any wound exudate noted on the dressing, this should be assessed and recorded, and reassessed regularly.

Activity

Check what the protocol is in your unit for wound care and postoperative removal of dressings.

The urinary catheter is usually removed at least 12 hours after the last dose of epidural anaesthesia, once the woman is mobile (NICE 2004). The trend in most units is to allow discharge home, if mother and baby are well, within 3–4 days, and no earlier than 24 hours postoperatively (NICE 2004). Women may need extra support at home, and part of good discharge planning should be advising her about the potential restrictions to her lifestyle such as driving, and most household tasks, especially heavy lifting, until the pain is no longer distracting or restricting (NICE 2004). Ongoing wound care includes observing for signs of exudate, dehiscence (separation of wound edges) or infection (NICE 2004).

Using best evidence

There is a range of evidence available on many aspects of surgical care for pregnant women, and this should be accessed to ensure you are providing best practice for your clients. For example, introduction of oral fluids and nutrition postoperatively is an important issue, particularly because good nutrition encourages effective wound healing. The main reason why midwives are cautious in reintroducing oral intake after caesarean is the risk of paralytic ileus, which is when there is lack of peristalsis within the ileum of the bowel, due to abdominal surgery. Research evidence does not suggest this is of particular concern in caesarean (Kramer et al 1996), and early reintroduction of oral fluid intake is also supported by a Cochrane review (Mangesi & Hofmeyr 2002). Consider too the other benefits of early reintroduction of food and fluids.

The Royal College of Obstetricians and Gynaecologists in association with NICE, have published the National Collaborating Centre for Women's and Children's Health's document *Caesarean section: clinical guideline* (NICE 2004). This summarizes all the available evidence on clinical aspects of care for caesarean section, and also evaluates the level of evidence available.

Safe environment

Immediately postoperatively the woman will be in the recovery area, usually for around 2 hours, where she can be closely observed. However, it is important to maintain her dignity and privacy, and balance this with your need to observe her. Keeping the curtains closed during examinations, bed baths, and infant feeding, can support this. Following this, the woman will be transferred to a postnatal ward, and the environment should be clean (to minimize infection risk), and easy for the woman to move around once

she is mobile. This may be a single room or a bed in a bay or ward with other women. Women who have had surgery need closer observation, and so often are placed in rooms nearest the midwifery 'station' on the ward, or in bays with similar women. Again, maintaining privacy is very important; curtains should be properly closed for all procedures and examinations.

Most importantly, the call bell should be kept within easy reach and should be working. Women who have had a caesarean have restricted mobility and independence and must be able to summon help without risking injury from falling out of bed or getting tangled in i.v. lines and catheter tubing.

Promotes health

In every aspect of care, you need to consider whether what you are doing promotes optimal health for mother and baby. Every aspect of the care you provide throughout the pre- and postoperative periods is a form of health promotion, by minimizing infection risk, promoting mobility and good mother–infant bonding, and by encouraging good nutrition, which contributes to maternal wellbeing and also improves wound healing. Mental and emotional health are promoted by supporting physical wellbeing as well as promoting the woman's independence whilst providing her with the right levels of support and practical help that she needs.

Other individual aspects of the care you provide might also contribute to health promotion. For example, it is recommended that all women are offered prophylactic antibiotics when undergoing caesarean section to reduce the risk of postoperative infections such as urinary tract infection, endometritis, and wound infection (NICE 2004).

Women having a caesarean should also be offered thromboprophylaxis as they are at increased risk of thromboembolism (NICE 2004). This includes use of anti-embolic stockings, good hydration, early mobilization and low molecular-weight heparin (NICE 2004). Anti-embolic stockings must be the right size, and women should have these fitted ideally prior to surgery.

Activity

Find out what the thromboprohphylaxis regime is in your unit. What form of low-molecular weight heparin is given, and at what intervals?

Team working

Surgical care involves liaison with a range of other professionals, throughout the whole perioperative period. The obstetric team will be consulted with on matters of clinical care and ongoing analgesia, wound healing and postoperative recovery, including, if necessary, suture or clip removal. Maternity care assistants can provide support with personal hygiene and infant care and feeding. Physiotherapists input on postoperative mobilization and deep breathing exercises which can help prevent postoperative complications such as deep vein thrombosis and pulmonary embolism.

Other professionals you might encounter include neonatologists and neonatal nurses, with whom you will need to liaise over infant wellbeing and care planning. A neonatal SHO should be present for all emergency caesarean sections, and for any case where there is any evidence of fetal compromise (NICE 2004). You will liaise with anaesthetists, operating department practitioners (ODPs),

porters, haematologists, and other theatre personnel such as the scrub nurse/midwife and the theatre runner.

Activity

Find out what care plans are in place in your unit.

Clinical dexterity

It is important to note the i.v. infusion and the rate, and to check the site of the i.v. cannula for patency and any signs of inflammation. This should be checked regularly, at the same intervals as the vital observations. The prescription chart should also be checked and the ongoing prescription for i.v. fluids noted. Any fluid restrictions should be noted and adhered to. Ideally, the intravenous infusion (IVI) should be running through an infusion pump set to the correct rate. Any i.v. fluids to be used should be checked against the prescription and checked with another midwife for contents and expiry date. The midwife should wash her hands, then close the roller clamp, remove the trochar from the old bag and insert it into the correct port in the new infusion bag. The roller clamp is then reopened at the correct rate. The fluid chart and prescription chart should be completed accordingly. PCA pumps should be checked, usually hourly, and the PCA check chart completed to monitor the amount of medication that has been used.

Fluid balance recording should be commenced on the correct form, and so the urinary catheter is also checked for patency, urine output and urine colour and concentration. It is important to properly care for the urinary catheter, which means minimizing the risk of ascending infection. It can be helpful to anchor an indwelling catheter with tape to attach it to the woman's thigh, to prevent traction from the bag or movement causing damage to the bladder (Boyle 2006). It is also important to position the catheter bag below bladder level, to keep it off the floor, and to clamp the tube when the woman is being transferred, again to minimize the risk of infection (Boyle 2006).

The midwife should check the abdomen for uterine tone and involution and check vaginal loss (usually at the same time as carrying out observations). Lochia may be heavier for women having caesarean section.

There may be a need to remove sutures or clips from the wound at a suitable time postoperatively. The timing of suture or clip removal can vary. For this, and for any invasive procedure, aseptic technique should be used (see Box 13.2).

Aseptic technique
An aseptic technique (see Box 13.2) should be used:

during any invasive procedure which breaches the body's natural defences, for example the skin, mucous membranes or when handling equipment which will enter a normally sterile area, urinary catheters or intravenous cannulae

(Xavier 1999:51)

Activity

Consider all the situations in midwifery practice to which the principle of asepsis could be applied.

Professional and legal
Midwives rules and standards (NMC 2004:10) states that 'the midwife must make sure the needs of the woman or baby are the primary focus of her practice'. This means that all of the woman's needs must be addressed, including surgical and other care and information needs. The midwife also has a responsibility to work in partnership with the woman and her family, enabling the woman to make decisions about her care based on her individual needs (NMC 2004:10). The NICE (2004) also state that 'pregnant women should be offered evidence-based information and support to enable them to make informed decisions about childbirth' (p7), including caesarean birth. Furthermore, the Code of Conduct (NMC 2008) states that midwives have a duty of care to provide safe and competent care. Therefore it is vital that all midwives develop the skills to care for women undergoing surgical procedures. Clients must, when giving consent for treatment, be legally competent and fully informed (NMC 2008). Consent should only be requested after women have been given evidence-based information, in a manner which respects the woman's privacy, dignity, views and culture, in the light of the clinical situation (NICE 2004).

Further scenarios

The following scenarios enable you to consider how specific situations influence the care a midwife provides. Consider the following in relation to the principles of surgical care.

Scenario 1

Delia has just been booked for an elective caesarean section due to placenta praevia.

Box 13.2 Procedure for aseptic technique

- **The dressing trolley should be cleaned daily with detergent and water or when physically contaminated and by alcohol wipes between use**
  Rationale To maintain a clean surface for sterile packs and prevent contamination between clients
- **Cleaning of the ward area and bed making should have ended at least 30 minutes before the procedure**
  Rationale To ensure any dust particles shaken into the air have had time to settle as they may fall onto an open wound
- **Bed curtains surrounding the woman should be closed at least 10 minutes before the procedure**
  Rationale To ensure any dust particles shaken into the air have had time to settle as they may fall onto an open wound
- **Wounds should be exposed for the least amount of time possible**
  Rationale To reduce the introduction of airborne organisms
- **Dirty dressings should be placed into an impervious disposal bag before leaving the bedside**

  Rationale To retain any micro-organisms and prevent cross infection by carrying them into the ward area
- **Clean wounds should be dressed before dirty ones on the ward**
  Rationale To prevent the cross infection of micro-organisms on trolleys or in the air that could be transferred to clean wounds
- **Windows should be closed, fans turned off and movement reduced around the area where the wound is being dressed**
  Rationale To reduce the airborne transfer of micro-organisms and keep the woman as warm as possible during exposure time
- **Handwashing should be carefully carried out**
  Rationale To remove micro-organsims and prevent cross infection between patients
- **The use of a non-touch technique by gloves or forceps**
  Rationale To prevent contamination with micro-organisms on the midwife's hands.

This is her first baby, and she is very concerned about the procedure, and its effects on her and her baby. She had been planning a home birth because she dislikes hospitals, particularly her local hospital because her mother died there recently, and she is very upset.

Practice point

Some women fear hospitals irrespective of their experience during pregnancy. The midwife needs to be able to identify how a woman is feeling and show compassion and caring when planning each individual woman's care. The woman's perception of her carer can have a lasting impact on how she perceives the birth.

Further questions specific to Scenario 1:

- How do you explain the caesarean section to her without causing further distress?

- How can you support Delia whilst ensuring she is fully prepared for the birth?
- What other measures can be taken to help Delia have a positive birth experience?
- Are there any resources that could be offered to Delia to help her adapt to her new role?

Scenario 2

You are looking after Sitta, who is about to have a Shirodkar suture inserted into her cervix. She is very nervous.

Practice point

Careful consideration needs to be given to women having cervical cerclage. Not only are they undergoing a surgical procedure but they are having it because they have previously experienced the effects of a cervical insufficiency and may be very fearful that they may also lose this baby.

Further questions specific to Scenario 2:

- What is a Shirodkar suture, what is it used for, and what is the procedure?
- How can you support and reassure Sitta?
- What observations must you carry out before and after the procedure?
- What ongoing needs will Sitta be likely to have, and how can you meet these needs?

- Who else might be closely involved in Sitta's care, and how will you communicate with them?

Conclusion

Providing care for women undergoing surgery is not only an important aspect of the role of the midwife, it is fundamental to meeting the needs of a range of women in differing circumstances, sometimes emergencies, in which stress and anxiety levels are high. Student midwives need to learn these skills and to develop and perfect them throughout their midwifery education programme, combining clinical aptitude with woman-centred, sensitive midwifery care. They need to work in collaboration with a range of different professionals and to draw on their expertise in ensuring that all the woman's needs, her baby's needs and her family's needs are met to the highest standards. This requires a good knowledge base, an understanding of safe practice, and the ability to communicate appropriately with all involved. Evidence and care standards exist to support midwives and their colleagues in the provision of this care, and provide guidance on all aspects of their role.

Useful resources

NICE 2004 Caesarean Section: Clinical Guideline. RCOG, London. Available online:
http://www.rcog.org.uk/resources/public/pdf/cs_section_full.pdf

Royal College of Anaesthetists guidance on the provision of obstetric anaesthesia services.

http://www.rcoa.ac.uk/docs/GPAS-Obs.pdf

Royal College of Obstetricians and Gynaecologists. Thromboprophylaxis green top guidelines.
http://www.rcog.org.uk/index.asp?PageID=535

References

Boyle M 2006 Wound healing in midwifery. Radcliffe Publishing, Abingdon

The Information Centre 2006 NHS Maternity Statistics, England: 2004–05. Community Health Statistics, London

Kramer R L, Van Someren J K, Qualls C R et al 1996 Postoperative management of caesarean patients: the effect of immediate feeding on the incidence of ileus. Obstetrics and Gynaecology 88: 29–32

Mallet J, Dougherty L 2000 Manual of clinical nursing procedures. Blackwell Science, Oxford

Mangesi L, Hofmeyr G 2002 Early compared with delayed oral fluid and food after caesarean section (Cochrane Review). The Cochrane Library Issue 3. Update Software, Oxford

National Institute for Health and Clinical Excellence (NICE) 2004 Caesarean section: clinical guideline. RCOG, London. Online. Available: http://www.rcog.org.uk/resources/public/pdf/cs_section_full.pdf. 25 May 2007

Nursing and Midwifery Council (NMC) 2004 Midwives rules and standards. Online. Available: www.nmc-uk.org. 30 May 2007

Nursing and Midwifery Council (NMC) 2008 The Code. Standards of conduct, performance and ethics for nurses and midwives. Online. NMC, London. Available: www.nmc-uk.org. 20 May 2007

Shah J L 2000 Postoperative pressure sores after epidural anaesthesia. BMJ 321: 941–942

Xavier G 1999 Asepsis. Nursing Standard 13(36): 49–53

Index